The Health Behavioral Change Imperative

The Health Behavioral Change Imperative

Theory, Education, and Practice in Diverse Populations

Edited and coauthored by

Jay Carrington Chunn

Morgan State University
Baltimore, Maryland

Kluwer Academic / Plenum Publishers
New York, Boston, Dordrecht, London, Moscow

Library of Congress Cataloging-in-Publication Data

The health behavioral change imperative: theory, education, and practice in diverse
populations/edited and coauthored by Jay Carrington Chunn.
    p.   cm.
  Includes bibliographical references and index.
  ISBN 0-306-47273-2
    1. Public health.   2. Health promotion.   3. Health behavior.   4. Medicine, preventive.   5. Mental
health promotion.   I. Chunn, Jay C., 1938–

RA427.8 .H475 2002
613—dc21

                                                                                        2002067823

ISBN 0-306-47273-2

©2002 Kluwer Academic / Plenum Publishers, New York
233 Spring Street, New York, New York 10013

http://www.wkap.nl/

10   9   8   7   6   5   4   3   2   1

A C.I.P. record for this book is available from the Library of Congress

Printed in the United States of America

Preface

The need for this book grows out of several realities: the deadly diseases that we collectively experience such as HIV-AIDS, sexually transmitted diseases, hypertension, diabetes, coronary heart disease, and stroke, among others, that are decimating communities of color. This stark reality constitutes a mandate for change. Additionally, the growing problem of violence in our society has reached pandemic proportions with a community such as Baltimore, Maryland experiencing over 300 homicides per year for the past ten years. That's over 3,000 young people primarily young black men between the ages of 16 and 26 being killed on the streets, with similar appalling numbers nationally in other urban areas. The growing reality of domestic violence, child abuse and neglect, and child sexual abuse occupy the public media all too often. The growing mass murders and the frightening spectacle of children killing children in their schools surely, in addition to the problem and madness enumerated above, demand that health professionals critically examine our health behavioral theories and prevention methodologies. Moreover, we are now challenged unlike any point in history to develop new theories and methodologies to deal with the above crisis. *The Health Behavioral Change Imperative*, indeed, exist, and we have a mandate to change behaviors that result in the deadly and crippling outcomes enumerated above.

Truly, we have embarked on the "third wave" of epidemiological reality where the most deadly diseases are not spread primarily by rodents, insects, or air/water born contaminates but by people in person-to-person contact, such as with HIV-AIDS spread by sexual and/or needle contact with infected persons. Indeed, the vast majority of the fatal and life-altering diseases we collectively face are preventable, however, only if our health behaviors radically change. *The Health Behavior Change Imperative is now in clear focus*. As discussed herein, health experts independently state that the most critical urban problems we face are preventable at a rate of between 95 and 98%. The resulting mandate is that a new breed of advanced public health practitioner needs to be trained as quickly and efficiently as possible capable of direct community based prevention practice in urban communities.

At Morgan State University, this author and the university recognized the critical need to educate and train a new breed "of public health professional" while at the same time eliminating a very significant societal contradiction and paradox. Until 1998, there was not one doctoral program in public health in any historically black college or university (HBCU), even given the alarming disproportionate presence of the critical health problems present in the black community and communities of color. The disparities in health status between black and white people as elegantly enumerated by the former Surgeon General of the United States, Dr. David Satcher, who consistently highlights across practically every health index disproportional morbidity and mortality in the black and hispanic community as enumerated in Healthy People 2000 (1998). In fact, HIV-AIDS is eight times higher in the black community and is four times greater in the hispanic community than in the white community which is a growing example of just one health disparity between the races.

In light of the above, this author prepared a prospective in 1996 setting forth the need to create the first Doctor of Public Health (DrPH) degree in a historically black college or university. The prospectus, as funded by the Kellogg Foundation, set forth the major tenants for the need for a creative four-year doctoral program designed to prepare doctoral level practitioners to impact urban communities with disease prevention services. Kellogg Foundation funded the planning effort and this author serves as the principal investigator for the planning effort. Hence, the need as addressed by Morgan's program to develop a new public health direct practice model for community-based intervention moved forward with considerable support. We are now at the end of the third-year operation of the DrPH program. The program was approved by the Maryland Higher Education Commission in December 1998 and admitted its first class of twenty-three doctoral (DrPH) students in August 1999 and admitted a like number in August 2000. Dr. Yvonne Bronner, from Johns Hopkins University, was hired in the summer of 1999 as director of the program and a talented faculty was recruited. The DrPH program at Morgan has established several centers as follows; HIV Prevention, Evaluation, and Policy Research Center, Morgan State University Cancer Prevention and Screening Center, the Center for Urban Public Health Policy, and the Youth Violence Prevention Center.

The author, from the beginning of the project, had an outstanding consultation-planning Group drawn nationally from a stellar group of public health professionals and governmental representatives. The nexus is, therefore, bridged and the contradiction and paradox noted earlier has been significantly impacted with the start of the DrPH and the MPH at Morgan. Thus, it became increasing clear to this author as the planning progressed that a new curriculum needed to be forged in full recognition of the behavioral aspects of our health crisis and the clear mandate for health behavior change and community based prevention. Thus, the concept of this book grew out of recognition that we must go beyond health education as understood and move to the core of behavior given internal locus of control issues and the non-feasibility of assigning responsibility for our health crisis totally on external agents and on racism although these are factors. In fact, the author and planning group of the DrPH program recognize that health behavior change is the primary objective of Morgan's program. This is the area where Morgan will excel and develop materials for others to utilize as well. Hence, the need for this book is validated and further work and development will be forthcoming out of the outstanding National Health Behavioral Change Task Force.

The ten chapters of this book confront the paradigm shifts and major transformation in the health arena from a public health perspective. The chapters are written from the public health perspective but have "planned variations" in primary themes and theory to allow the reader to have several strategies; this book to be utilized with different communities of color and universally as well. Further, innovative concepts are advanced that support rebuilding the black community-village as a nurturing and supportive place for young people to grow and develop. The chapters challenge the reader to place faith and its healing power into an interactive process along with new insights into the theory from a comparative theological perspective given the twelve-step programs as a viable and penetrating response to communities plagued with chronic addictions and its attendant behaviors. Other chapters consider prevention as an emerging science, and several chapters present prevention and health behavior change as a process and product which must be responsive to color and culture. In so doing, the chapters forge collectively toward a new public health practice behavioral perspective while developing and discussing theory and conceptualizations designed to impact positively a new community-based advanced public health practice. This book may therefore be utilized as a textbook in schools of public health and programs in psychology, social work, counseling, and in related disciplines where behavior change is crucial to survival and the wellness process. This book importantly recognizes the paradigm shifts and societal-health care transformations that are redefining public health, medical care, and health services delivery practices. Thus, a foundation is potentially forged, given societal transformations, for creating wellness and not only treating disease as the primary goal and not the continued maintenance of "sick care" (Chissel, 1999) as health's primary mission. Indeed, our greatest challenge is in the prevention of disease and maintaining wellness as advanced through out this book by all of the chapters and authors.

JAY CARRINGTON CHUNN

Acknowledgments

The deepest gratitude and indebtedness is owed to all of the authors who contributed to this book. Without their unselfish and steadfast efforts and contributions this work would not have come to fruition and completion. The chapters contained within this book were commissioned by the editor and all written specifically for this publication. Further the content was further refined in a special Symposium called by this author in the Summer of 1999 attended by an interdisciplinary audience of forty experts from psychiatry, psychology, social work, counseling, governmental service and community based health organizations. The Symposium was called because the author wanted to take our collective scholarship, theories and applications to the "market place" as in Plato's Academy to engage in discourse regarding the critical issues raised by each chapter. Each of the chapters herein was presented in the two day Symposium and rewritten given the rich discourse with experts that transpired and transformed these works within the "market place". As you recall in Plato's Academy, on a daily basis, the scholars would convene in the market place and share their ideas and theories with the public in discourse. This process provided invaluable peer review, cross validation and additional input into the notions and theories advanced. The Symposium was video taped in its entirety and can be made available to practitioners and others upon request at a reasonable cost.

The Kellogg Foundation funded the Symposium and publication efforts from the planning grant for the Doctor of Public Health degree program Master of Public Health (MPH) (DrPH). The new doctoral program was fully implemented in August 1999, enrolling twenty-three full time students. The MPH program was implemented a year later in 2000. President Earl S. Richardson of Morgan State University and other key administrators supported the planning effort with enthusiasm; staff and faculty of the University remain supportive. Dr. Bailus Walker, a former President of the American Public Health Association, was hired as the planning director-consultant to assist this author and Principal Investigator in planning and preparing the full proposal for the Maryland Higher Education Commission review. Vice President Clara I. Adams remained enthusiastic and supportive of the planning process from the initial discussions to the present and has been most helpful in assisting the implementation efforts. Special appreciation is extended to Dr. Henrie Treadwell, Kellogg Foundation Program Officer, for her unrelenting support of our efforts and for her creativity and confidence in this author and respect for Morgan State University in recommending the $264,000 planning grant. Dr. Treadwell remains very much supportive of our public health initiatives at Morgan State. The same appreciation is extended to Rosalyn Brock for her enthusiastic support as my past program officer. Also the help of Tamra Fountaine, administrative assistant to Ms. Brock, has been most supportive and enabling in completing the planning process. The funds for the excellent

Health Behavioral Change Task Force, which diligently worked for four years prior to the publication of this book, also came from the Kellogg grant. The work of the Health Behavioral Change Task Force for the last four years culminated in these chapters. Thus, their expertise, competence, skillful writing ability, and dedication to improving the health status of people of color and others continues to be self-evident.

The Consultation-Planning Group that advised during the planning effort for the DrPH and MPH degree programs are also extremely talented and dedicated and served with great distinction during the degree-planning effort. Most attended every meeting and traveled to Baltimore from as far away as Texas and other locations. They represented the best universities in the world in our program planning being from the Public Health Schools of Johns Hopkins University, Harvard University, the University of North Carolina and, the University of Texas in Austin among others.

The members of the Planning Group were all outstanding respected leaders in public health practice and education that continue to be leaders in the public health practice in their respective Schools of Public Health. Importantly, we also were blessed to have in our planning group representatives from the Office of Minority Health, The Center for Disease Control/Registry for Toxic Waste Administration, and the former health policy expert of Congressman Louis Stokes' staff. We were also blessed to have the Commissioner of Public Health for the State of Maryland and the Deputy Commissioner of the Baltimore City Public Health Department as a member. Special appreciation is extended to Dr. Clay Simpson, former Director of the Office of Minority Health and Deputy Assistant Secretary of Health (HHS) who gave this author the first and most valuable consultation in 1996 with seasoned wisdom along with his full and enthusiastic advice to proceed. Dr. Simpson remarked on the uniqueness of the seamless four-year doctorate within the prospectus; his advice provided, at that stage of the beginning process, the cross-validation needed to encourage this author and our collective program planning efforts. He also stated that for years he had wanted to have a Public Health doctoral program in a historically black college or university.

This author would also like to acknowledge the support and encouragement of Morgan State University staff and faculty who gained knowledge about this project and offered help and encouragement. Special thanks are extended to my secretary Emily B. Henry for her assistance during the planning of the academic programs and through the activities that culminated in this book. Special thanks are extended to several doctoral and advanced students and my doctoral interns with whom ideas were shared about the DrPH program and this book over the past three years. Special appreciation is extended to former intern Dr. Beverly O'Bryant, who served as a reader and editorial assistant for Dr John Wheaton. Their encouragement and input has proven quite helpful and insightful. Profound and special appreciation is extended to those that served at various times as assistant editors, first and second readers, and word processors such as Constance Mann. Special praise and thanks goes to Publishing Director Mariclaire Cloutier and Assistant Editor Teresa Krauss for their encouragement and enthusiasm regarding this book.

Finally, the editor and co-authors thank and acknowledge with the deepest appreciation the help and support and ongoing encouragement of our family members, colleagues, and significant others. Without their patience and understanding, this book would have been most difficult to produce. To the readers of this publication, the editor acknowledges responsibility for any technical errors that remain.

Contents

Chapter 1

**The Health Behavioral Change Imperative: Paradigm Shifts and
Prevention Mandate** **1**
Jay Carrington Chunn

Chapter 2

Strategies for Health Behavior Change **17**
Carl C. Bell, Brian Flay, and Roberta L. Paikoff

Chapter 3

Cultural Competence in Behavioral Health Care **41**
Derald Wing Sue

Chapter 4

**Prevention Science: Theory, Research, and Implications
for Practice** **51**
Warren A. Rhodes, Rolande Murray, and Marlene Greer-Chase

Chapter 5

Violence Prevention in African American Youth **61**
William R. Lawson, Jimmy Cunningham, and Valerie Lawson

Chapter 6

**Applying Mental Health Behavioral Change to
Ethnonational Conflict Resolution** **73**
Maurice Apprey

Chapter 7

**Development of Authenticity in Public Health: A Culturecology
Model as a Culture Critique** **91**
Lewis M. King

Chapter 8

**The Preparation and Scope of Practice for Future Advanced
Public Health Practitioners in Doctoral Programs** 113
Rena G. Boss-Victoria

Chapter 9

The Social Context for Faith and Health 127
Rueben C. Warren, Harold C. J. Lockett, and Adrian A. Zulfiqar

Chapter 10

**Healing an Addiction through a Twelve Step Program
Ending in Faith** 153
George Laney, Gregory E. Rogers, and Ricky Phaison

The Coauthors   171

Index   173

The Health Behavioral Change
Imperative

Chapter 1

The Health Behavioral Change Imperative

Paradigm Shifts and Prevention Mandate

JAY CARRINGTON CHUNN

A Challenge for the New Millennium

The public health community and general public collectively face a crisis of major proportions. Diseases such as HIV-AIDS, sexually transmitted diseases, cancer, strokes, coronary artery disease and others have grown in morbidity and mortality and render high-risk populations at the greatest vulnerability in history. In the case of AIDS, while the death rate is decreasing due to more effective medications such as protease inhibitors and azidothymidine, those infected are still victims of eventual death. The reality of the vast morbidity and mortality that we face precipitates a greater search for prevention. We now know and understand that HIV-AIDS, sexually transmitted diseases, drug abuse, alcohol abuse, and most other urban health problems are preventable.

Over the past three years in all of this author's major speeches and presentations to health audiences, comprised of medical doctors, public health workers and health knowledgeable professionals, surveys were conducted using focus group techniques to solicit dialogue and responses on urban health problems. From a national review of health and medical literature and in discussion with health professionals, the following priority areas in urban health were identified:

Priority Problem Areas in Urban Health

- HIV-AIDS
- Substance Abuse
- Mental Health
- Coronary Artery—Heart Disease

- Child/Adolescent Health
   Cancer
   Breast
   Prostate
   Lung
- Suicide
- Smoking
- Violence
   Interfamilial
   ○ Domestic Violence
   ○ Child Physical and Mental Abuse and Neglect
   ○ Sexual Abuse
   External
   ○ Homicide
   ○ Robbery
   ○ Assault
- Sexually Transmitted Diseases (STDs)
- Diabetes
- Hypertension

These diseases and health problems are not listed in a prioritized manner. The audiences, which were utilized partially as focus groups, include representatives from the Psychiatry and Behavioral Science Section of the National Medical Association, The Public Health Symposium Group conducted by this author at Morgan State University, The Association of Black Hospital Pharmacists, in addition to HIV-AIDS prevention audiences comprised of psychiatrists, psychologists, social workers, nurses, health care administrators and community-based (CBOs) public health practitioners. The critical question posed to these groups over the past three years was, "Of the above critical health problems in urban communities what percentage of these problems are behaviorally based and preventable?" After much thoughtful discussion, the consensus of all the groups stated 95 to 98 percent. Prevention, therefore, is the key to improving the heath status in urban areas where high-risk populations are primarily located. The populations are at higher risk due to the interaction of factors, including race, gender, socio-economic status, educational level and related variables.

The trends that are developing nationally are reflected most graphically in Baltimore. In March 2000 it is reported by the HIV Surveillance Office (Baltimore City Health Department, 2000) that Baltimore, extrapolating from earlier data, most likely has the highest HIV prevalence rate among U.S. cities. Further, in 1996–98, Baltimore was ranked as number one (1) in syphilis in the country and this year, 2000; it is reportedly ranked number two (2) in syphilis.

In Baltimore City it is estimated as follows:

- Approximately 18,000 residents of Baltimore City are believed living with HIV-infection:
   ○ 5,000 living with AIDS
   ○ 7,000 HIV positive, tested, and identified to the local health authority
   ○ 6,000 HIV positive, not tested, or tested prior to 1994 or not identified to the local health authority

- Women continue to be the fastest growing group of new infections and AIDS cases
  - Women make up the largest portion of those untested and unreported
  - HIV infected women experience *Pneumocystis carin* pneumonia 1.4 times more often than men
  - Maryland has the fifth highest number of children living with AIDS in the U.S.
- Drug Abuse is a factor in approximately 90% of new AIDS diagnosis
  - IDU or other substance abuse issues have a role in all new pediatric HIV cases
- Baltimore City is home to 60% of all new HIV infections in Maryland, with only 12% of the population
- The leading cause of death among 25–44 year olds in Baltimore City has been HIV since 1989
- The decline in the AIDS Case Registry has ameliorated on a quarter-by-quarter basis
- A number equal to 1.7% of Baltimore's current population has been diagnosed with AIDS since 1981
- Extrapolating from earlier data, Baltimore likely has the highest and/or among the highest HIV prevalence rate among U.S. cities
- 6,100 Baltimore AIDS cases have died since the epidemic began (Baltimore City Health Department, 2000).

Figures 1–3 graphically illustrate the crisis in Baltimore City.

Figure 1 illustrates the change from a much higher white HIV positive rate to the convergence between races in 1991–1992 and the current disparity between the races with a much higher rate among blacks.

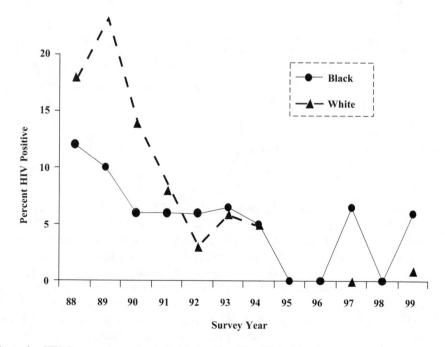

Figure 1. HIV Seroprevalence among Baltimore City STD Clinic Clients by Race, 1988–1999 (*Source:* Baltimore City Health Department; HIV Surveillance, March, 2000).

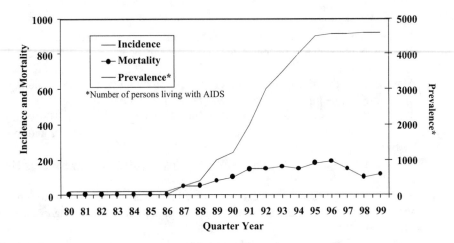

Figure 2. AIDS Incidence and Mortality vs. AIDS Prevalence City of Baltimore, Maryland on Two Scales through Second Quarter, 1999 (*Source:* Baltimore City Health Department; HIV Surveillance, March, 2000).

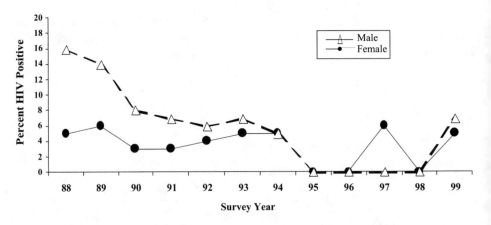

Figure 3. HIV Seroprevalence among Baltimore City STD Clinic Clients by Sex, 1998–1999.

The prevalence rate noted in Figure 2 reflects the 18,000 residents in Baltimore City living with HIV infection. Note, however, the mortality rate continues to decline.

Figure 3 notes the convergence of male and female seroprevalence, which really highlights the heterosexual nature of HIV changing from a primarily male-dominated homosexual phenomenon to now involving both sexes almost equally.

Baltimore's experience with HIV infection is instructive for the nation. Baltimore currently has over 60,000 drug addicts and only approximately nine thousand treatment slots. The trading of sex for drugs is well known among addicted persons, as is the sharing of needles. Cities with high addiction rates face the same escalating dangers. Also keep in clear focus the reality that sexually transmitted diseases (STD) serve as markers for HIV infection with a continued high correlation between STD's and HIV infections. Baltimore is currently number (2) in syphilis. Further, drug addictions in the prisons along with high HIV infection rates continue to cause major problems as prisoners' transition back to the community. Bisexual individuals are involved and have sex with men and also sex with women without disclosure of their bisexuality. This phenomenon helps to explain the higher rate of prevalence between Black women of childbearing age.

It should also be noted that bisexuality is more prevalent in society than homosexuality. However, it is not disclosed readily in the Black community. This is most likely an intervening variable in the almost identical HIV seroprevalence rate between males and females in Baltimore as noted on the charts. The health behavioral change mandate is even more clearly focused given the above. It is not just Baltimore that is impacted by this high prevalence rate, but neighboring cities and states given the mobility of the public. The contributing factors to this HIV crisis must be handled with more treatment slots, person to person interventions, more prevention programs that use effective theoretical-based strategies, and health behavioral change strategies that are effective.

The Paradigm Shifts in Health Care

Given the above realities of the diseases, especially HIV-AIDS, that have negative impact on the health status of urban populations, these realities place a disproportionately higher risk upon Blacks, Hispanics, and others. These diseases are preventable, and mandate a shift in foci of intervention regarding our medical and health care practices. Hence, the *Health Behavioral Change Imperative is in clear focus.* We must work diligently and vigorously on society's practice to only treat disease and shift this priority to the prevention of disease. This mandate has several components, including a nexus of issues on the practice level including those of health care, health delivery, and health and environmental policy. Again, the mandate of the *Health Behavioral Change Imperative* is clear: We *must nationally focus our efforts on disease prevention!* This will prove most profitable in human terms, both in the saving of lives and in improving the quality of life for millions of people. From a cost control basis, it is less costly to prevent disease than to pay for its health-and-life-destroying consequences. The multi-billion dollar tobacco claim settlements across the United States clearly illustrate this reality. Maryland alone will receive a settlement of $5 billion over the next 20 years.

Careful analysis of the most critical health areas that we face discussed above, especially as related to HIV-AIDS and sexually transmitted diseases, reveals the rapid infecting of urban and populations of color, given vaginal, oral and/or anal sex, and the sharing of drug needles that transmit the HIV virus. The paradigm shifts reveal that HIV-AIDS is not airborne, nor externally transmitted by an unknown agent; it is transmitted by person-to-person sexual or person-to-person needle contact. This reality, then, makes it even more critical that we must immediately give more emphasis to the social and behavioral sciences to develop effective health behavioral change strategies.

This paradigm shift also mandates a change in the way we approach high-risk population groups and communities. The traditional approach utilized by medical and public health and preventive-community health practitioners' focuses on the professional being the primary agent in an "acting upon" modality. Hence, the health professionals are imposing from above the intervention with the client/patient and community in a passive, recipient posture. *Within this paradigm shift the most effective approaches to health behavioral change entail the individual taking responsibility for the behavioral change and closely involving the family and community components to positively reinforce the behavioral change strategy.* This is critical because we must identify the factors in the individual's immediate environment that can assist in changing the behaviors, rather than conceding any ground to high-risk sexual activity, drug and/or alcohol abuse, violent behavior as well as nutritional and diet-related issues and similar variables. Research on substance abuse and alcohol-related disorders point to poly-drug abuse rather than to a single destructive agent. Sexual dysfunction, as well as nutritional and diet deficiencies and complications quickly follow. Individuals taking responsibility for their own health behaviors will ensure a longer and more effective behavioral change outcome than by proceeding differently.

Another paradigm shift further reveals a most critical reality. There is a vast disconnect between what we know will destroy or negatively impact our health and lives, and how we subsequently behave. The disconnect is growing even wider, for modern science and scientific diagnostic tools reveal now more than ever the danger in our individual and collective behaviors, hence, the paradigm shift is from personal and social lack of knowledge on disease etiology to gross denial of behavioral realities and consequences. For example, we now know that having multiple sex partners and engaging in unprotected sex places us at greatest risk for HIV-AIDS. Even though ninety seven percent (97%) of African Americans know this, we still have morbidity in this area at eight times the rate within the White community, and four times the rate in the Hispanic community (Kaiser Survey, 1998). We are also informed by the same survey data that ninety one percent (91%) of pregnant women with HIV-AIDS know that they can infect their baby, and that seventy three percent (73%) know there is no cure for AIDS. These examples show that knowledge alone of the deadly and harmful impact of the disease does not significantly change the behavior. Hence, the *behavioral disconnect* is obvious with HIV-AIDS, as it is with smoking behaviors, drug abusing behaviors and similar issues. Smoking behavior points to psychological gross denial, for the Surgeon General, Dr. David Satcher, warns that smoking may cause heart, lung, and related diseases, and this is clearly printed on each cigarette pack! In fact, the packs also say that each cigarette causes carbon monoxide poisoning. Therefore, given the above, we must confront the *behavioral disconnect* on both individual and on societal levels. On the individual level we must therefore utilize social and behavioral sciences change interventions, and on the societal level, we must use social policy and planning, social marketing, and environmental prevention strategies.

Increasingly, survey data reveals readiness of the African American community to utilize and implement societal environmental change information and methods. The paradigm shift emphasizing person-individual causal agent(s), being most instrumental in spreading the new wave of infectious diseases as discussed earlier, is creating readiness of African Americans to seek more information, knowledge and change strategies (Kaiser, 1998). For example, sixty two percent (62%) report that they want more information on what to discuss with kids about HIV-AIDS prevention; fifty five percent (55%) want to know where to go for help if exposed; forty six percent (46%) want to know more about testing for HIV. Consistently, communities seek more information on what to discuss with partners about sex with forty percent (40%) wanting more general information, and with twenty seven percent (27%) wanting more knowledge on the proper way to use condoms. The data strongly suggest both readiness for intervention, and also, importantly, the possibility for meaningful and, we hope, long-term health behavioral change. Further, we must now recognize, given the totality of the survey results and by the disconnect between what is known and is behaviorally carried out, that warnings in health education do not alone prevent high-risk behaviors.

The paradigm shift of the private physician-patient relationship (usually maintained in a solo or small group practice) to managed care is very significant. Factors that contribute to this paradigm shift include rapidly escalating cost of care, which implies that managed care is perceived as much cheaper than private or small group practice. Individual medical practitioners alone cannot make decisions on course of treatment or methodology without a "business" decision by a "manager of cost," external to the managed care clinic. Hence, due to rapidly escalating cost, seven to nine years ago, managed care was viewed and continues to be viewed by many as the most effective cost control method. This, according to most physicians, continues to be a major factor with an impact yet to be determined, for it allegedly implies unnecessary interference in the doctor-patient relationship, and therefore hinders quality medical care. Many physicians have complained to this author that in working for managed care systems they have only 15 minutes to see their patients, which is too short for them to provide quality care. This debate continues and must await longitudinal studies that document quantitative differences in morbidity and mortality data in comparative studies with traditional medical practice. The qualitative differences are surely obvious, as illustrated within each system that is preferred by doctor or patient.

Notwithstanding the previous discussion of managed care, it is generally accepted that to make managed care work, a relatively healthy population is desirable and required. Hence, prevention becomes of the highest importance so that managed care agencies will have an opportunity for success. Managed care systems, with too many sick and aging people who require costly treatment and therapies, will go bankrupt quite rapidly. This is certainly the case in Maryland, where seven out of ten managed care systems have imploded within the last three years because of cost factors, and have gone out of business. Aggressive prevention work is required through public and patient education, early and thorough patient diagnosis, and assessment and early intervention for health problems that may lead to more disease and more costly treatment.

Health care in America must shift health and medical systems from primarily only treating illness to health promotion and disease prevention. Hence, this paradigm shift rejects illness as our major focus of health care, to recognition of wellness as the optimal condition. Therefore, preventing illness is of the highest priority. In fact, we have in this country a sick care system, not a health care system (Chissel, 1997 and 1999). A health care system would reinforce wellness, the care of individual, and family health. This seems so logical and easy to understand; it is therefore amazing that we are primarily equipped to treat sick people, and not to prevent people from getting ill. Dr. David Satcher, Former Surgeon General of the United States, speaks to the fact that we spend over a trillion dollars a year on treatment of disease, but spend only about 1.4 percent of that on prevention (Satcher, 2000). Changing this reality will take a major effort, including critical public policy and health policy refocusing, as well as increasing awareness in pubic health graduates (masters/doctorates) and changing the way they are trained. Public health graduates should emerge with advanced practice skills and knowledge, in addition to competence in research and epidemiology. *This reality further highlights the primary need in public health for practitioners to be educated and trained to engage in community-based prevention practice, working directly with* communities.

This does not preclude these graduates, as discussed above, from having strong research and epidemiological strengths. *Further, this crucial paradigm shift and redirection will also call for very significant changes in medical education of physicians, equally emphasizing how to prevent disease, and how to provide alternative medical care, thus focusing on a wellness philosophy.* This paradigm shift does not preclude this newly trained and refocused medical doctor from being as skilled in diagnosis and treatment; however, the physician will have new dimensions in his or her philosophy of practice, with emphasis on wellness, not just on disease. For example, in speeches and presentations at national health conferences, this author regularly asks that psychiatrists, physicians and health professionals expand their thinking, and consider how they would prevent, with early intervention, each of their patients from having the presenting medical problem they observe in their practice. They are asked to assume that they could treat their patients prior to any symptom occurring.

How would doctors ensure that their patients remain asymptomatic, and/or would not have the illness at all? The answer lies in using medical knowledge of disease and treatment to create wellness rather than exclusively for treatment of disease! Similar shifts in emphasis will also be required by our leading health systems and hospitals, forcing them to focus more on wellness and community interventions. Thus, they would have to seek strategies and partners to maintain healthy neighborhoods and devote more of their revenue and resources to the areas of prevention, community medicine, and prevention practices.

The preparation of public health practitioners will also have to go through radical change, and must produce practitioners at both the masters and doctorate level. The first model of this kind requiring a continuous four-year course of study at Morgan State University in Baltimore, Maryland was originally conceptualized by this author. The program enrolled its first class of doctoral students in August 1999 and they will emerge as *advanced prevention practitioners* in 2003. This innovative program will be discussed much later in this chapter.

A paradigm shift increasing in momentum and reality is the merging of community-based hospitals and health care systems with like institutions and teaching hospitals to compete more successfully for market share. A major factor in this paradigm shift is improved medical care and treatment techniques; resulting in shorter hospital stays, and managed care limiting the number of days stay in hospitals. Cost and revenue generation are essentially the driving forces propelling this paradigm shift. Many smaller, mid-size hospitals and health care systems cannot remain competitive, and must merge with larger systems to survive. The larger hospitals, health care systems, and university teaching hospitals are often initiating these mergers to move their operations closer to communities and community-based practice to further expand their market share. Hence, they are also recognizing in the controlling of cost that effective care must utilize economy of scale and also maintain a healthier population. These factors are equally compelling because of quality of life issues and cost-containment issues that, given this shifting health care reality, constitute a nexus of realities that must serve and respond to a paradoxical set of factors.

There is an increasing awareness among many in the health care field that we are moving incrementally, but deliberately, into a posture where universal health care for all Americans is in the realm of possibility for the future. The latest development in this area is a congressional proposal under review, which would pay for all prescription medication for the elderly. Forty-four million Americans are without health care insurance, and aren't acknowledged until they flood emergency rooms. *The use of emergency room resources as a physician service by the uninsured calls for and demands a paradigm shift to universal health care. The neglect of uninsured populations is also evident in the billions of dollars being spent for uncompensated care in this country, which has a negative impact on local, state and institutional budgets.* This reality is leading to the trend of placing the uninsured and under-insured into managed care operations in return for Medicare and Medicaid dollars as well as tax revenue dollars. This provides a fragile financial support structure. This is a challenge, because these uninsured populations are often much less healthy than the general population. This author's cost-benefit analyses reveal, however, that it is cheaper per capita to serve this population through managed care than to continue the out-of-control cost of uncompensated care. The reality of serving chronically under-served populations within managed care is leading to the failure of many managed care agencies. Moreover, managed care cannot be successful with low income, chronically ill populations due to the increased cost burden as previously discussed. Hence, prevention is of vital importance in maintaining and making profitable managed care agencies.

The last paradigm shift noted in this chapter is the move of focus from internal-self with emphasis on individual illness and personal frailties, to external self-with emphasis on environmental and societal policy and practices influencing individual and group health. This paradigm shift is noted in increased emphasis on environmental policy regarding brown-fields, air-ground-water pollution, industrial and radioactive waste, public smoking bans, and raising cost of cigarettes, liquor and in similar issues. These issues are recognized as major public policy, and practice issues and are being addressed by State Legislatures and Governors, as well as the year 2000 presidential candidates. President Clinton and Congress have collectively given close attention in 1999 to environmental public policy and factors that influence community and individual health.

The recognition of the powerful impact of smoking is complex. Factors such as the freedom of choice issue (internal locus) must be augmented by consideration of advertising deceit and corporate manipulation, along with the illegal practice of intentionally adding addictive substances to tobacco products (external locus). The tobacco industry does this to create long-term dependence on smoking. Also, the horrid practice of intentionally marketing to children and young people, primary in communities of color among Blacks and Spanish-speaking people, creates a new generation of tobacco-victimized customers and is the primary environmental external locus of control issue. The reverse sides of these arguments are realities, as previously discussed, of having 95% to 98% preventable urban-based diseases. Therefore, we must take responsibility for our health behaviors and recognize the *behavioral change imperative* as presented in this book. This reality is not only tolerated but moves to the heart of the cost nexus along with the quality of life questions raised in this chapter. This paradigm shift recognizes the interwoven nature of

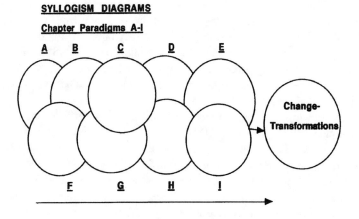

Figure 4.   Paradigm shifts.

behavioral, biological, genetic, cultural, familial and environmental factors in disease etiology and outcomes.

The paradigm shifts, as noted in Figure 4, create momentum and pace of change, which are constant in a dynamic and not static society. The paradigm shifts move forward in an exponential manner as illustrated in the natural sciences due to advances and innovations in science and the health care community. The sum total of these and other paradigm shifts discussed in this chapter, and resulting changes create the transformations taking place in health care and in health care policy. Hence, the change and momentum of change created by the paradigm shifts continue to foster the massive transformations we are experiencing in public health and health care. These transformations will continue well into the 21st century, and will eventually radically change public health practice, medical practice, health policy, patient care and health services delivery systems.

Health Behavioral Change Theory and Practice Dimensions

It is now generally accepted that if we can reduce and eventually eliminate high-risk behaviors, then we will greatly impact the rate of new HIV-AIDS infections, tobacco use, drug use, sexual behaviors, injury, and other health problems. The Center for Disease Control and Prevention (CDC) in 1997 concluded a national school-based Youth Risk Behavioral Survey that received 16,262 questionnaires completed by students in 150 schools (CDC, 1997). Among the risk behaviors that worsened were tobacco use, drug use, sexual behaviors and reduced rates of physical activity as noted in Figure 5.

African Americans continue to represent the highest risk group for new HIV-AIDS infections representing approximately forty-seven percent (47%) of all new cases. It is further recognized that African American women of childbearing age are the fastest growing population group with new HIV-AIDS infection. HIV infections are also on the increase with the older population, age 50 and beyond. A recent NIH research report, (1998) revealed that behavioral interventions significantly reduced HIV-AIDS related sexual risk behaviors.

The National Institute of Mental Heath (NIMH) Multisite HIV Prevention Trial enrolled 3,706 men and women in 37 inner-city clinics. A seven-session intervention based on motivation and skills significantly reduced several sexual risk variables over a one-year period of time. STD's were reduced during the period of intervention. The study utilized seven sites in five urban areas. Study participants were drawn from men and women in public STD clinics, and from women utilizing primarily public health care clinics. Racial group analysis of the subjects revealed that sixty-eight percent (68%) of subjects were African American and twenty percent (20%) were Hispanic. All were at high risk for HIV infection. The study revealed behavior change with cognitive and behavioral social science interventions over the seven-session intervention.

There is a growing body of evidence on the effectiveness of behavioral change interventions in reducing the high risk of HIV-AIDS, drug abuse, and related behaviors. These interventions are carried out at the community level, and show considerable promise, especially in regard to prevention of HIV infection. The CDC conducted a study focused on community level intervention to encourage progress toward consistent condom and bleach use among high-risk HIV populations in five major cities (Fishbein, 1999). Behavioral theory was the primary intervention, utilizing role-model stories, which were distributed with condoms for sexual activity and bleach for use on needles. Community members

	1991	1993	1995	1997
Tobacco use				
Current cigarette use[2]	27.5	30.5	34.8	36.4
Frequent cigarette use[3]	12.7	13.8	16.1	16.7
Drug Use				
Current marijuana use[4]	14.7	17.7	25.3	26.2
Lifetime cocaine use	5.9	4.9	7.0	8.2
Lifetime illegal steroid use	2.7	2.2	3.7	3.1
Offered, sold, or given an illegal drug on school property[5]	NA	24.0	32.1	31.7
Sexual behaviors				
Used birth control pills at last sexual intercourse[6]	20.8	18.4	17.4	16.6
Physical activity				
Participated in vigorous physical activity[7]	66.3	65.8	63.7	63.8
Attended physical education class daily	41.6	34.3	25.4	27.4

Figure 5.   Youth Risk Behavior Trends: Risk Behaviors that Worsened,[1] 1991–1997.

[1] Significant linear change, $p < .05$; [2] Smoked cigarettes on >1 of the 30 days preceding the survey; [3] Smoked cigarettes on >20 of the 30 days preceding the survey; [4] Used marijuana >1 time during the 30 days preceding the survey; [5] During the 12 months preceding the survey; [6] Among currently sexually active students; [7] For at least 20 minutes on >3 of the 7 days preceding the survey. NA: Data not collected.

encouraged behavioral change among injection drug users and their sexual partners, both female and male. This approach recognizes the importance of culture and environment in treatment and in maintaining the gains made in treatment.

The study found that the intervention resulted in significant community-wide progress toward consistent HIV-AIDS risk reduction. Hence, the research theory nexus regarding social science use in prevention reinforces the concept of paradigm shifts, and the need for wellness strategies and programs as we experience the transformations taking place in the public health and health care industry. Community-based behavioral change strategies must have impact on users and individuals by actively involving them in the process, bringing patients and clients "to the table" as decisions and policy are formulated.

In addition to behavioral theory and cognitive theory, social learning theory holds considerable promise for affecting health behavioral change. This theory and resulting practice builds on models based on people understanding the effects of personal and environmental dynamics on their health behaviors. Social learning theory holds two approaches, one with a behavioral approach and the other cognitive. Individuals with an internal locus of control appear to be healthier than those who have perceived external controls (Richman et al., 1982; Wallston, 1981; Strickland, 1979). Preventive health habits, proper diet, dental hygiene, proper exercise, and regular medical checkups have been demonstrated to transfer to health habits later in life according to Lau (1982). There is a growing body of research pointing to much healthier behaviors such as smoking cessation (Strickland, 1978; Wallston and Waiston, 1982) utilizing social learning and other theories.

Bandura's research and concept of self-efficacy (1977) speaks to beliefs and convictions that individuals have what they need to carry out behaviors required to produce desired outcomes. These expectations have a direct influence on options and choices that people make. This is compelling in that social cognitive theory encompasses the external environment and its capacity to reinforce and/or negate behavior. Research by Kalichmen, Carey and Johnson (1996), focused on HIV risk reduction interventions based on social learning theory that examined sexual behavioral change, which was determined to be quite effective. Further research by Early (1996) regarding condom use utilized social learning theory and intervention, which was shown to be effective when compared with a non-use control. This approach holds considerable promise to help people overcome destructive health behaviors because it takes into account factors unique to the individual, and social-societal factors as well. This author predicts considerable use of this theoretical and practical approach, along with social learning theory, given the increased funding for smoking cessation programs and with the substantial funding levels resulting from tobacco settlements.

Other theoretical models also hold promise for health behavior change, such as the Health Belief Model, which partially explains the failure of people to participate in various programs designed to prevent as well as discover disease (Hochbaum, 1958; Rosenstock, 1960, 1974). This model helps to explain how people react to disease and illness (Rosensock, 1990). The theory of reasoned action also holds much promise in that it predicts a person's intention to perform a behavior based on intent (Fishbein, 1967; Fishbein an Ajzen, 1975, 1980). Attitudes and the social environment are critical factors; a person's values and belief system enter as determinants of attitude. This model also takes into account cultural factors that influence attitude and, in a broad sense, incorporate elements of social learning theory in determining behavioral outcomes. This theory should prove more and more effective in dealing with sexual behaviors that could lead to sexually transmitted diseases and HIV-AIDS. Given also this model's sensitivity to cultural and environmental factors, it should also prove more and more effective in treating alcohol and drug abuse, as these behaviors are strongly reinforced by cultural factors and peer pressure. The nexus between intent and culture is critical in addictive behavior as evidenced in the example of differences within Black and Hispanic cultures in which interventions must be culturally sensitive. This is documented and discussed in other chapters within this book.

The use of a transtheoretical model of change has many uses against many behavioral health issues, including violence. This approach deals with stages of changes, with self-efficiency and decisional process both interlocking, and reinforcing each other (Prochaska, 1983; Grimley, 1993). This approach offers a model that moves a person through stages, from pre-contemplation, contemplation, preparation, action, maintenance, and relapse. What is extremely promising about this approach is that the interventions move parallel to the stages of change. These interventions range from persuasive communications, information, to how to show development and reinforcement, support and self-management. Thus, there is a series of interventions, depending on the stage of behavior change. This model, developed principally by Prochaska (1994) with contributions by Bradley-Springer (1996) and Grimley, Riley, Bellyard and Prischeski (1993) is applicable to widely disparate behaviors from alcohol and drug abuse, violence, to sexual behaviors and smoking cessation, for which it was originally developed.

A behavior change strategy with great promise, but one that is greatly underutilized is social marketing. In our society we use marketing techniques and methods to move products, goods, and services. Advertisers have the methods and technology to sell practically anything—from cars, houses, toothpaste and clothing to every commodity produced in this country and in a world economy. Marketing not only sells but also creates demand. Advertising and marketing also tell consumers when to change products, or to trade-in an old product for a newer model—often long before the older model is obsolete.

If such impact on behavior is possible with manufactured and produced goods, why is *behavioral* change not possible with *social* marketing given that we sell cigarettes by marketing. The public health profession should challenge social marketing to use the same techniques and strategies to bring about smoking cessation. It can be done. The same outcome is true for alcohol and drugs of abuse, for which we create images of sexuality to sell and promote with great sophistication. We should therefore, conversely, create negative imaging for smoking and abuse of alcohol and drugs. Anti-violence campaigns could also be waged using mass media, like marketing is used to create demand for new products. The present public service announcement methods will not work, because they employ only a few announcements, late at night, or early in the morning when fewer people are watching.

We must spend as much money on social marketing that is used to create and maintain mass consumption of goods and services that society produces and purchases. The annual Super Bowl Football Classic is a prime example. Major companies pay up to $40 million for a three-minute commercial with beer being the most frequently advertised product. The same amount of emphasis and prime time exposure is required to market anti-smoking, anti-drinking and anti-violence messages. It is hypocritical at best for the company with the highest advertising budget to sell alcohol products—and then, place a six-second message at the end to: "use alcohol wisely" or similar message after $40 million have been spent on three minutes of all the glitz and glamour possible in today's television technology. Surely a society with America's wealth can afford to protect its children, youth and families from this type of exploitation that uses hype to persuade them to consume alcohol and cigarettes!

It must be stressed that the theoretical approaches discussed in this chapter must be adjusted, as appropriate, given the reality of people of color and the impact of culture on behavior and health determinants and health outcomes. Not any one theory or theoretical model designed for one cultural group will fit the needs different from its own. This is of special significance given the differences noted by race, culture and eco-environmental factors unique to each group. Hence, there is no "magic bullet" theory, but more research is needed in order to impact and extract theory and application relevant to people of color. Given where we are, however, we must move quickly with this agenda while at the same time adjusting existing theoretical notions and models, many of which are presented in these chapters, to meet our collective needs.

Closing Discussion

Health behavioral change is a nationally mandated imperative. It actually speaks to the heart and soul of our quality of life, life expectancy and longevity, and to the survival of a large segment of our society. The current pandemic we are experiencing with HIV-AIDS is illustrative of our current reality. Baltimore, Maryland, for example has experienced approximately 10,000 AIDS cases since 1981. As of April 2000, 5,000 of these AIDS patients survive. More alarming, Baltimore currently has 18,000 HIV infected persons (Baltimore City Health Department, 2000). It has been recognized that HIV infected persons may experience as many (average) as ten sexual partners each. If this holds true in Baltimore, then approximately 180,000 of its citizens may be at risk—a full one-third of the population. This dismal reality is made even graver by the realization that Baltimore has over 60,000 active drug addicts, and only approximately 9,000 treatment slots. This translates to approximately 50,000 addicts having to resort daily to illegal means to get and stay high. Sex for drugs and needles for drug sharing has become a dangerous reality. The Baltimore community is now number one nationally according to the City Health Department with HIV-AIDS in proportion to its population (City Health Department, 2000). Baltimore was number one in syphilis two year ago, and in the top five for gonorrhea and related diseases (CDC, 1998). Problems with similar dimensions exist in other cities like New York, Washington, D.C., San Francisco, and other urban locations. We are experiencing the largest and most deadly health crisis in the modern history of this country.

The good news is that the health problems that continue to dominate many of our urban and inner-city communities are preventable. The bad news is that society and individuals have not accepted the challenge to practice prevention and reallocate resources for that purpose. As discussed at the beginning of this chapter, analysis of focus groups surveyed by this author reveal that 95% to 98% of the urban health problems including all of the sexually transmitted diseases, such as HIV-AIDS, are all preventable according to health care experts. We are the disease agent and the carrier; therefore, we have to change our behaviors and take responsibility for what has happened. The solution is obvious, but what is lacking thus far is the individual and collective will to bring about change. Change must take place along a continuum, from individual behavior to family group, community, public, economic, and social change.

Incremental change is frustrating, and does not feed the transformations in health care that the profound paradigm shifts are forcing as quickly as needed. These changes, however, are vitally important as they move the health politic forward. Transformations in public health and health are taking place that signal new potential. The tobacco settlements are one such example with billions of dollars being made available over the next twenty or more years that can be used for improving the health status of millions of Americans. Our hopes are that significant amounts of the tobacco money are being allocated for prevention. It is very important now, more than ever, that public health take a strong advocacy position to ensure that the tobacco settlement dollars are not politically used in "pork-barrel" projects, but in many ways that speak to primarily tobacco-related diseases, such as cancer and heart disease. Maryland is attempting to focus its funds primarily for cancer treatment and smoking cessation in spite of some political moves by several legislative members to practice "pork" as usual. The Governor, however, remained locked on course, advocating cancer treatment and smoking cessation. With approximately $60 million available to Maryland this year, only a small percentage (less than 10%) is earmarked currently for prevention. This is not enough, and defies the paradigm shifts and resulting transformation in public health and health care that are taking place.

The debate about placing 90% of available smoking dollars into treatment and not prevention begs an ethical and policy question to focus on those affected, but does very little beyond tokenism to prevent others from having the same affliction. The resolve of this ethical and policy dilemma is to strike a balance between treatment and prevention. Moreover, public health must take on a more active and politically aggressive advocacy role to ensure the additional funds needed for prevention.

At Morgan State University, this author had the pleasure and honor of conceptualizing the first doctor of Public Health degree program at a Historically Black University (HBCU). The Kellogg Foundation funded, the planning effort in 1996, with this author being the Principal Investigator. The degree was not conceptualized to carry out business as usual. The doctoral program was conceptualized to prepare a generation of new public health practitioners. These new specialists operate from a community-based prevention perspective with the ability to intervene, prevent and solve problems such as HIV-AIDS, STD's and to help others to reduce high morbidity and mortality rates from cancer, diabetes, strokes and other societal factors that precipitate these illnesses. The new practitioner is prepared to practice far ahead of the paradigm shifts and transformations impacting urban communities. The public health profession as currently documented is primarily training practitioners to practice in the old paradigms, and prepares their graduates for traditional research and assessment roles.

The new practitioner being prepared at the doctoral level at Morgan will have the opportunity to graduate in four years after earning the bachelor's degree and will emerge with special prevention skills in working with urban high-risk populations with the most vexing health and violence problems (Chunn, 1983). Thus, within a reasonable number of years, (five to eight) Morgan will graduate a critical significant mass of predominantly Black practitioners with skills to make a major impact on how public health is practiced. They will be empowered to really make a difference in the quality of life in high-risk communities. Therefore, a new Doctor of Public Health practitioner will have skills that are useful on the block, in the neighborhood, community, city, and state as well as on federal levels, along with systems change and prevention intervention modalities. The model can be replicated at other colleges and universities as several have made contact to make visits or request materials for the purpose of starting their own programs (Appendix—Chunn, 1995).

Further, the community-based practitioner will also have strong research skills along with epidemiological skills to further advance community-based practice; and, a scientific basis for intervening, coupled with solution-based theoretical and practical knowledge. Our reality and society demand that we actively confront the hard issues of transformations discussed in this chapter. The Health Behavioral Change Imperative is directional, and much needed to ensure a healthier future for the urban dwellers and families. We must prepare for the transformations ahead of the paradigm shifts, and provide the required leadership to enhance the quality of life for those in the greatest need. The mandate is clear. Let us accept the mandate and challenges ahead, and forge a new community-based primary prevention practice model, as well as practitioners at the doctoral level who are equipped and trained to have positive impact on health-related behavior change.

References

Bandura, A. (1977). Self-efficacy: Toward a unifying theory of behavior change. *Psychological Review*, 84, 191–215.

Bandura, A. (1977). Social learning theory. Englewood Cliffs: NJ: Prentice-Hall.

Baltimore City Health Department. *HIV Surveillance Project*. March 2000.

Bradley-Springer, L. (1996). Patient education for behavior change: Help from the transtheoretical and harm reduction models. *Journal of the Association of Nurses in HIV-AIDS Care*.

Chissel, John (1999). The health behavior change symposium sponsored by Morgan State University, June 1999. Funded by Kellogg Foundation, Baltimore, Maryland.

Chissel, John (1993). *Pyramids of power: An ancient African centered approach to optimal health*. Baltimore, MD: Positive Perception Publication.

Center for Disease Control and Prevention (1997). *Youth risk behavioral survey, National school based with 150 schools*. Atlanta, 6A: CDC.

Center for Disease Control and Prevention (1998). *National school based youth risk behavioral survey*. Atlanta, 6A: CDC.

Chunn, J.C., Dunston, P.J., and Ross-Sheriff, F. (1983). *Mental health and people of color: Curriculum development and change*. Washington, D.C.: Howard University Press.

Fishbein, M. (1967). Attitude and the prediction of behavior: Results of a survey sample. In M. Fishbein (Ed), *Readings in attitude theory and measurement*. New York: Wiley.

Fishbein, M. and Ajzen, I. (1975). *Beliefs, attitudes, intention and behavior: Introduction to theory and research reading*. Reading: MA: Addison-Wesley.

Grimley, D., Riley, G., and Balin, J. (1993). Assessing the stages of change and decision making for contraception: Use, prevention of pregnancy, sexually transmitted. *Health Education Quarterly*. 20.

Kalichmen S. Carey, M., and Johnson, B. (1996). Prevention of sexually transmitted HIV infection: A meta-analytic review of the behavioral outcome literature. *Analysis of Behavior Medicine*. 18, 6-D.

Lau, R. (1982). Origins of health locus of control beliefs. *Journal of Personality and Social Psychology*. 42, 322–334.

Osborne, O., Carter, C., Pinkieton, N., and Richards, H. (1987). Chapter 13: Development of African American curriculum content in psychiatric and mental health nursing. In J.C. Chunn, J.P. Dunston, Ross-Sheriff's *Mental health and people of color: Curriculum development and change*. Washington, D.C.: Howard University Press, (1983).

Prochaska, J. and DiClemente, C. (1983). Stages and process of self-change of smoking: Toward an Integrative Model of Change. *Journal of Consulting and Clinical Psychology*. 5, 390–395.

Prochaska, J. and DiClemente, C. (1984). *The transtheoretical approach: Closing the traditional boundaries of therapy*. Homewood, IL: Dow-Jones/Irvin.

Prochaska, J., Reading, C., Harlow, C., Rossi, J., and Veficer, W. (1994). The trans-theoretical model of change and HIV prevention: A review. *Health Education Quarterly*. 21, 471–486.

Prochaska, J., Reading, C., Harlow, C., Rossi, J., and Veficer, W. (1994). *The trans-theoretical model of change and HIV prevention*.

Kaiser Family Foundation (1998). *National survey of African Americans and HIV-AIDS*. March.

Rosensock, I. (1990). The health belief model: Exploring health behavior through expectance. In Glanz, Lewis Reimero (Eds), *Health behavior and health education: Theory, research and practice*. San Francisco: Josey Bass.

Satcher, D. (2000). *Eliminating disparities in health: The surgeon general's prescription*. Speech delivered at Morgan State University on February 3, 2000, in celebration of the first year of the Doctor of Public Health Degree Program by Dr. David Satcher, Surgeon General of the United States and Assistant Secretary of Health, Department of Health and Human Services. Baltimore, Maryland.

Wallston, K. and Walliston, B. (1982). Who is responsible for your health?: The construct of health locus of control. In G. Sanders and J. Suls (Eds), *Social psychology of health and illness*. Hillsdale, NJ: Lawrence Erlbaum.

Chapter **2**

Strategies for Health Behavior Change

CARL C. BELL, BRIAN FLAY, AND ROBERTA PAIKOFF

Introduction

Currently, the major risks to health are the result of engaging in risky behavior. Risky behaviors include not seeking treatment for psychiatric disorders, engaging in unsafe sex, escalating interpersonal conflicts, and abusing drugs. The authors have been involved with two research projects and one large-scale naturalistic study—all of which underscore several key principles necessary to cause a health behavior change. Accordingly, we will highlight and explain these principles to guide future prevention/intervention initiatives designed to improve the health of under-served populations. The seven field principles that we will highlight are: (1) rebuilding the village, (2) providing access to health care, (3) improving bonding, attachment, and connectedness dynamics within the community and between stakeholders, (4) improving self esteem, (5) increasing social skills of target recipients, (6) reestablishing the adult protective shield and monitoring, and (7) minimizing the residual effects of trauma.

The Chicago HIV Prevention and Adolescent Mental Health Project (CHAMP)

Currently, Drs. Paikoff (Principal Investigator), McKay (Co-Principal Investigator), and Bell (Collaborator) are involved in an HIV prevention research project aimed at reducing the incidence of HIV infection in an area of Chicago with higher than average city wide seroprevalence rates [Other co-investigators include B. Carlvin, M. Culps, M. Hewitt, E. McKinney, L. McKinney, F. Oden, (Beethoven School); D. Baptiste, D. Coleman, G. Coleman, I. Coleman, J. Fuller, S. Madison, A. McCormick, S. Parfenoff, R. Scott, L. Wright (CHAMP); S. Sewell (CMHC); E. Bowers, M. Ellis, D. Phillips, D. Thompson, B. Turner, D. Wade, and L. Williamson (Coleman School); B. Easter, G. Nash, D. Nolan,

(McCorkle School); P. Hughes and J. Matthis (Faraday School); E. Fleming (Taylor Park); S. Boyd, B. Scott, D. Shaw, and A. Thrasher-Johnson (Terrell School); M. Davis (Westside), S. Simmons (Community parents).]

In this area are the Robert Taylor Homes, a Chicago housing development with several thousand, poor and underserved African American residents and their children. Because Robert Taylor community individuals are at high risk for getting HIV, Drs. Roberta Paikoff and Mary McKay developed the Chicago HIV Prevention and Adolescent Mental Health Project (CHAMP) originally piloted to work on HIV prevention with African American 4th to 7th grades at a Chicago Public Grammar School on the Westside. The project developed a curriculum for parents from Robert Taylor to deliver, in partnership with University of Illinois mental health interns, aimed toward Robert Taylor children who attend four Chicago Public Grammar Schools in the community. The curriculum was developed based on: (1) basic developmental research with children and families on the South and West Sides of Chicago (Paikoff, 1995, 1997), (2) principles of multiple family group delivery and engagement in family programs (Tolan & McKay, 1996); (3) literature on prior successful behavior change programs (Jemmott, Jemmott & Fong, 1992; Szapocznik, 1996); and (4) extensive community collaboration over time (McKay, Baptiste, Coleman, Madison, Paikoff & Scott, 2000; Madison, McKay, Paikoff & Bell, 2000)

The curriculum teaches students, parents, and families issues related improving: (1) parenting children, (2) monitoring children's behavior, (3) improving the connectedness between parents and their children, and (4) increasing parental support by connecting parent with one another to function as mutual support systems. In addition, we focus on the health behavior risk of unsafe sex. Therefore, we seek to increase HIV prevention knowledge and to foster attitudes and family communication regarding these issues during children's pubertal development. Further, we discuss family values on dating and sexuality, and the family role in child assertiveness and refusal skills.

The project is a true academic/community partnership, with the governing board consisting of both academic and community board members who run the project. After the University of Illinois gets its indirect cost off the top, the other funds are split 50/50 between the academics and the community participants. As a collaborator on this project, Dr. Bell provides leadership that builds the spirit of collaboration between the stakeholders (Madison, McKay, Paikoff & Bell, 2000).

ABAN-AYA

Drs. Flay (Principal Investigator) and Bell (Co-principle Investigator) [Other co-investigators include: Shaffdeen Amuwo and Judith Cooksey (School of Public Health), Julia Cowell and Barbara Dancy (School of Nursing), Sally Graumlich and Susan Levy (Health Research and Policy Centers), Robert Jagers (Departments of African-American Studies and Psychology), Roberta Paikoff (Department of Psychiatry and Institute for Juvenile Research), Indru Punwani (Department of Pediatric Dentistry), and Olga Reyes and Roger Weissberg (Department of Psychology, University of Illinois) are involved with the Chicago African-American Youth Health Behavior Project (Aban-Aya)]. This project is a public school-based community effort addressing violence, drug use, and inappropriate sexual behavior prevention, and is housed in the Health Research and Policy Centers (HRPCs) of the University of Illinois at Chicago.

This project maintains a more traditional research structure of principal investigators and co-investigators providing the leadership for the intervention, and project staff providing the actual day-to-day intervention work. Beyond funds paying the investigators and project staff is a smaller budget set aside for community members who work part-time assisting in the intervention.

There are three conditions in this health behavior change research project: (1) an Afro-centric health education control, (2) an Afro-centric social development curriculum (SDC) aimed at violence, drug use, and inappropriate sexual behavior, and (3) the SDC with a community development component. The SDC involves increasing students' self-esteem, social skills, attachment to the schools, and information about health behavior risks. The SDC community condition additionally seeks to augment the community partnerships and reestablish the adult protective shield along with monitoring. This project is large and involves sixteen different school sites in the Chicago area.

The design of the interventions was informed by the Theory of Triadic Influence (TTI) (Flay and Petraitis, 1994) that provides an integration of multiple sociological and psychological theories of behavior and behavior change. The TTI incorporates sociological theories of social control and social bonding (Akers et al., 1979; Elliot et al., 1985), peer clustering (Oetting & Beauvais, 1986), cultural identity (Oetting & Beauvais, 1990–91), psychological theories of attitude change and behavioral prediction (Fishbein & Ajzen, 1975; Ajzen, 1985), personality development (Digman, 1990), social learning (Akers et al., 1979; Bandura, 1977, 1986), and other integrative theories (e.g., Jessor & Jessors, Problem Behavior Theory; Brook's Family Interaction Theory, Hawkins' Social Development Theory). See Petraitis, Flay and Miller (1995) for a review of many such theories.

The TTI (Figure 6) includes five tiers of causes of behavior that range from very proximal to distal to ultimate, and three "streams" (and 6 substreams) of influence that flow

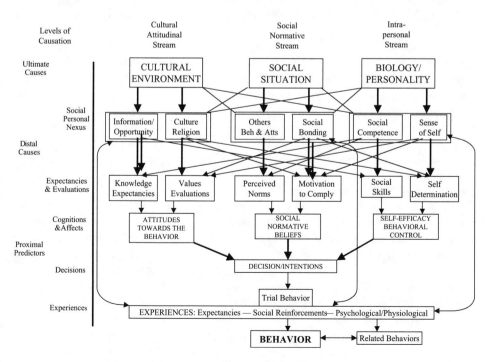

Figure 6. The Theory of Triadic Influence.

through the seven tiers. (1) cultural-environmental influences on knowledge and values →
attitudes; (2) social situations' contextual influences on social bonding and social learning →
normative social beliefs; and (3) interpersonal influences on self-determination/
control and social skills → self-efficacy.

In addition to the direct influences of these streams, there are important inter-stream
effects and influences. The theory is intended to account for factors that have direct and
indirect effects on behavior—both new and regular. Experiences with related behaviors and
early experiences with new behavior lead to feedback loops through all three streams,
adding to the prior influences of these streams. This integration of existing theories leads to
a meta-theoretical view that suggests higher order descriptions and explanations of health
behavior, that, in turn, suggest new approaches for health promotion and disease prevention.

Chicago Board of Education Violence Prevention Initiative

Finally, Dr. Bell has been consulting with the Chicago Board of Education about violence
prevention. In 1998, the Chicago Public Schools (CPS) revealed its violence prevention
initiative that originated from the central office. The seven field principles found in this
initiative, which are also found in the previous two projects, are (1) rebuilding the village,
(2) providing access to health care, (3) improving bonding, attachment, and connectedness
dynamics, (4) improving self-esteem, (5) increasing social skills, (6) reestablishing the
adult protective shield increasing monitoring, and (7) minimizing the residual effects of
trauma.

The purpose of this contribution is to underscore the seven field principles that are
necessary for any successful universal health behavior intervention. Though TTI contains
these seven field principles and is a useful comprehensive theoretical construct upon which
to develop health behavior interventions, it may be too complicated to be used for guidance in the field.

Using the above public health prevention/intervention efforts, the authors will discuss
the seven field principles of: (1) rebuilding the village consisting of developing and
expanding community partnerships and coalitions (a broad sociocultural influence that
entails a level of community organization around health behavioral issues-"cultural/attitu-
dinal stream" and "social/normative stream" of TTI, (2) providing access to health care
(addresses highly influential, individual-level risk factors that require a community-level
service—"biology" in the intrapersonal stream of TTI). (3) improving bonding, attachment, and connectedness dynamics within the community and between stakeholders
("social bonding" in the social/normative stream of TTI), (4) improving self esteem
("sense of self" in the intra-personal stream of TTI), (5) increasing social skills of target
recipients ("social skills" in the intra-personal stream of TTI), (6) reestablishing the adult
protective shield and monitoring problem behaviors ("others' behavior and attitudes" in
the social/normative stream of TTI), and (7) minimizing the residual effects of trauma
("behavioral control-self-management skills and affect regulation" in the intra-personal
stream of TTI). As we have described the efforts by CHAMP, Aban-Aya, and the Chicago
Board of Education elsewhere (Madison, McKay, Paikoff & Bell, 2000; McKay, Baptiste,
Coleman, Madison, Paikoff & Scott, 2000; Paikoff, 1997; Smith et al., in press; Bell,
Gamm, Vallas, and Jackson, 2001; Flay and others, work in progress), rather
than give details of the programs, we will highlight them as examples of the seven field
principles.

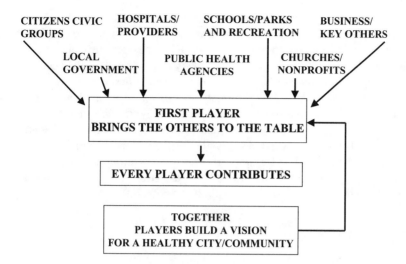

Figure 7. Any player starts. (*Source*: Adapted from: *Healthy People in Healthy Communities: A Guide for Community Leaders*. U.S. Department of Health and Human Services, Public Health Service, Office of Public Health and Science, Office of Disease and Health Promotion, June 1998).

Developing and Expanding Community Partnerships and Coalitions

Several years ago, Dr. David Satcher, former U.S. Surgeon General, once asked "How do you deliver public health interventions in communities that lack infrastructure?" After thinking about his question for a year, our answer was that there had to be a facilitator that helped the community develop infrastructures by initiating community partnerships and coalitions. Figure 7 illustrates this process. This figure illustrates how one player—any player—brings the other players to the table to build a vision of a healthier community.

CHAMP

In CHAMP, the players who brought the other players to the table were a developmental psychologist (Dr. Roberta Paikoff), a Ph.D. social worker (Dr. Mary McKay), and community advisors at six Chicago Public schools who wrote a grant to attempt HIV prevention in Chicago's Robert Taylor Homes. These researchers had the foresight to recruit a facilitator (Dr. Bell) to guide the university/community collaboration in developing an egalitarian model of collaboration (Hatch et al., 1993; Madison, McKay, Paikoff & Bell, 2000). Specifically, the community members were to progress from advisors to full collaborators. They were to participate in the direction and focus of the research. As full collaborators, the community members were to have a role in the conception, implementation, and interpretation of the research.

In addition, a basic principle of the CHAMP intervention was to help families collaborate to form mutual support groups. By families pooling resources to monitor children, the children are safer from engaging in high-risk behaviors associated with contracting the HIV virus. The program was based on both intervention and developmental literature about HIV primary prevention, and general principles of human sexuality. Most programs traditionally have aimed primary prevention at high school youth, who are likely to be sexually active already (e.g., programs aimed at delaying the onset of sexual behavior): Youth who are already sexually active are far less likely to be sexually influenced by such programs than are youth who are not yet sexually active (Miller, Card, Paikoff, & Peterson, 1992; Howard & McCabe, 1990; Jemmott & Jemmott, 1998). Therefore, the goal of CHAMP was to involve youth before an initial onset of sexual behavior. In a series of studies of youth's understanding of their sexual behavior, youth have consistently reported more contextual, rather than individually- based facilitators of early sexual experience (Paikoff, 1995; Paikoff and others, work in progress). Therefore, we almost aimed the program at changing contexts by providing child assertiveness training and refusal skills (McKay, Baptiste, Coleman, Madison, Paikoff & Scoff, 2000).

ABAN-AYA

In the Aban-Aya project's SDC/community intervention, we developed local school task forces to develop collaborations with the community. In this instance the principal investigator (Brian Flay) provided leadership for the Aban-Aya co-investigators, the project coordinator, and health educators to become players who brought other community players to the table. The purpose of the local school task forces was to increase parental and community involvement in the day-to-day activities of the school and to be supportive of Aban-Aya efforts. There is evidence that school-based interventions that shift how they manage high-risk children can reduce risk for in-school violence (Elliot & Tolan, 1999). Increasing parental involvement in school and increasing parental and community collaboration can accomplish this with school personnel (Comer, 1988; Haynes & Comer, 1996; Haynes, Comer, & Hamilton-Lee, 1989).

Chicago Board of Education Violence Prevention Initiative

The Chicago Public School strategy involved partnering with community-based secular and non-secular organizations to foster activities designed to reduce violent and disruptive behavior by and against youth in the school and surrounding communities. We designed these partnerships to share the vision of a violence-free environment. In this instance the player who brought the other players to the table was the leadership of the Chicago Board of Education (C.E.O.: Paul Vallas, Chief of Staff: Philip Jackson, and Specialized Services Coordinator: Sue Gamm). By partnering with the religious community in the "CPS Interfaith Community Partnership," CPS could increase attendance, improve school environments, provide positive role models, and create activities for youth. At present, it provides support to twelve religious school-community partnership networks in each of the CPS regions. This partnership-coordinated anti-violence marches with religious communities throughout the city. In addition, the network of secular organizations provided assistance in mentoring programs, off-site detention and community service programs, and assistance with after-school homework centers. Further, there was a "Walking-Men School Bus" that recruits men to escort children to and from school.

Besides these efforts, CPS initiated efforts to partner with the community by developing the "CPS Youth Outreach Workers" program that they started during the "Safe

Schools, Safe Neighborhoods Summer" 1998 Initiative. This effort trained 100 Violence Intervention Program Specialist compromising off-duty police, community members, parents, teachers, and social workers to provide positive alternative activities for youth in high crime areas. Also, they created a referral service network that reported and provided follow-up services for more than 2,000 referrals for suicide risk, recreational activities, job preparation, job orientation, job placement, gang detachment, and housing relocation issues. The CPS youth outreach workers' efforts facilitated collaborative partnerships with more than fifty governmental and city agencies and community-based organizations.

CPS also developed many school-community activities, especially for schools whose communities experience high rates of violence. An example is the CPS Englewood Youth Violence Prevention Program, a community-based plan to reduce crime and violence for three schools in the West Englewood community. This program's intervention and prevention activities included efforts designed to ensure that youth comply with curfew laws and provided intervention with gang members to reduce gang activity. The program also offered tutoring, family strengthening services, and social services.

Another example is the CPS Logan Square Neighborhood Association (LSNA). The goal of this effort was to create up to five community-learning centers to serve families in adult education, children and youth education, and recreational programming. In addition, the association provided homework assistance, childcare, and other family-focused activities. LSNA has trained more than 400 parents, who are then placed in classrooms where they tutor children and help the teacher.

There are several other community councils and alliances consisting of local churches, community organizations, residents, schools, and law enforcement that are helping parents to: (1) coordinate violence prevention activities of parents themselves, (2) hire and train parent patrols and parent attendance officers, and (3) develop evening sports programs. These efforts increase safety of students, parents, school staff, and increase attendance and learning environment. We see another CPS effort at developing community partnerships in the CPS Region anti-Violence Workshops. These summer regional workshops, address violence issues affecting school and their surrounding communities. Through collaborative relations with the Local School Councils and the Chicago Police Department's Community Action Policing (CAP) they have identified and distributed program community resources.

Although all three projects made efforts to get various players at the table, getting players at the table is just the first step of developing collaboration. Another major consideration is each player's role in the collaboration. Hatch et al. (1993) proposed four models of collaboration: (1) where community representatives, who may or may not be community residents, are involved to give advice and approval, (2) where influential community representatives are involved as advocates of the intervention's efforts, (3) where community members may have jobs on the intervention as advisors but who do not provide any leadership for the intervention, and (4) where community members provide leadership for the intervention by developing a model, starting the intervention, and interpreting the outcomes. By emphasizing the shared vision a facilitator can encourage a mission-driven philosophy. Such a philosophy encourages diverse elements within society to attach to the mission, and place it above fewer important driving forces, e.g., "egos" or "turf."

The question is: How does a partnership become a true coalition? Our experience is that by emphasizing the ecological relationships between diverse elements in a community, a good facilitator can encourage attachment/affiliative/approach behaviors between these various elements. Further, emphasizing the ecological relationships encourages the development of systems thinking. By providing leadership to the diverse community elements, the facilitator encourages religious, business, social service, health, educational, civic, social, and other organizations to participate in an assessment of the nature and size of the problem. Thus, CHAMP stakeholders sized the problem of HIV, Aban-Aya stakeholders measured the problems of violence, drug abuse, and inappropriate sexual behavior, and Chicago Board of Education assessed the problem of school violence. The reader can obtain much more information about this process from the web site http://ahecpartners.org.

Clearly, communities with social fabric have less "deviant behavior" due to the prevention of this behavior (Sampson et al., 1997). Shaw and McKay (1942) proposed the social disorganization theory of deviance suggesting that few job opportunities, poverty, single-headed households, isolation from neighbors, and weakened community friendship networks and community institutions lead to reduced, informal, and formal social control. Elliot and Tolan (1999) note community organization efforts are producing promising results, although applying traditional scientific criteria to community organization experiments is difficult.

Health Care

This principle addresses highly influential, individual-level risk factors that require a community-level service. Individuals' needs sometimes overwhelm any intervention and must be attended to.

Moffitt (1997) gives ample evidence that neuropsychiatric factors impinge on behavior. There is evidence children with high exposure to lead may be predisposed to violence (Bell, 1997b; Earls, 1991). Further, there is evidence children who have Attention Deficit Hyperactive Disorder (ADHD) may be predisposed to violence and conduct disorder (Klein et al., 1997). This disorder may predispose children to engaging in other high-risk behaviors such as drug abuse or early onsets of sexual behavior (American Psychiatric Association, 1994). Finally, evidence that neuropsychiatric disorders may predispose individuals to violence exists (Lewis et al., 1985). Clearly, to promote health behavior change in individuals with these psychiatric or behavioral disorders, treatment for neuropsychiatric disorders is essential. As neuropsychiatry becomes more sophisticated, the causes of impulse control problems will become more specific. In addition, as neuropsychiatry evolves, psychiatric treatment of impulse control problems that cause risky behavior will become more specific. For example, we are constantly discovering more specific treatments for drug addiction (American Psychiatric Association, 1996). Without developing the diagnostic and service delivery infrastructure to provide these more sophisticated services, communities with the greatest need will be the last to receive appropriate health care that can prevent some causes of risky health behaviors.

CHAMP and ABAN-AYA

Except for providing referrals when the need arises, CHAMP and Aban-Aya do not specifically seek to increase access to health care of their research subjects. While such efforts are beyond the scope of these two focused research projects, an increased access to health care is clearly a value of the researchers and program staff of these two projects. Consequently,

CHAMP provides linkages to health care services, and a comprehensive resource directory to all participating families. CHAMP developed the directory through collaboration between social work interns and community partners, and updates it annually.

Guerra (1997) notes two categories of prevention programs: state and locally funded service programs and university or research group supported research programs. She further observes that both service and research programs face problems with implementation. Service programs can be more flexible, while research programs lack this flexibility and are often more focused on specific research questions. Thus, CHAMP and Aban-Aya are required to study particular aspects of the health behavior change paradigm, while service-based prevention programs in the Chicago Public School can be more encompassing.

Chicago Board of Education Violence Prevention Initiative

Because Chicago mandates that the Chicago Public schools educate children who have psychiatric or behavioral disorders, CPS have stepped up efforts to ensure children have access to primary health care and social service to promote healthy social and physical development. Accordingly, CPS developed Healthy Kids/Healthy Minds. This service provides free hearing aides and eye examinations for under- and uninsured students. They also provide dental screening and cleaning for all elementary students. These efforts have established links between 300 schools and social service and health agencies.

As a pilot school-based outreach program of the U.S. Department of Education, CPS is collaborating with community health agencies and the Illinois Department of Public Aid to expand the number of eligible children and families for Medicaid and public insurance in a program called Kid Care. Expanded coverage enables children greater access to school-community health and social services.

Bonding, Attachment and Connectedness Dynamics

Bowlby (1973, 1988) and Ainsworth (1973) theorized that failure to form a secure attachment with caregivers during infancy has a strong influence on peoples' ability to form trusting relationships later in life. Meloy (1992) provides ample evidence that individuals lacking in secure attachments during infancy may later form violent attachments resulting in chronically violent relationships. Similarly, Renken et al. (1989) found youth who engaged in aggressive behaviors were the most insecurely attached to their families. Several researchers' observations confirm the fact that low levels of parental warmth, acceptance, and affection, low levels of cohesion, and high levels of conflict and hostility have been associated with delinquent and violent behavior (Farrington, 1989; Henggeler et al., 1992; Tolan & Lorion, 1988). There is also evidence that aggressive children show more "insecure" attachment styles (Booth et al., 1992). Further, there is an association between delinquency and weak attachment bonds to parents (Hirshchi, 1969). Eron, et al., (1991) found that parental rejection was strongly related to youth's later criminal outcomes. Similarly, research has shown that low levels of parental warmth, acceptance, and affection, low levels of cohesion, and high levels of conflict and hostility are associated with children who engage in early sexual behavior (McBride & Paikoff, 1999).

Fortunately, early intervention (i.e., from ages 0 to 3) can improve problems with attachment. Sroufe, Egeland, and Kreutzer (1990) find that many children change attachment classifications throughout the first few years of life; thus, there is malleability of attachment relationships over time. Urie Bronfenbrenner (1979) has also written about the potential importance of attachment figures outside the family, where familiar attachments are not secure. Pinderhughes (1972) outlined the importance of attachment behaviors in violence prevention and intervention efforts. Further, empirical studies reveal family variables of children being connected to their parents and school variables of being connected to the school are associated with reduced risk taking (Resnick et al., 1997). In addition, Borduin et al. (1985) notes that improving intra family relations—closeness, positive statements, communication clarity, and emotional cohesion—can reduce risk for serious antisocial behavior and violence. Alternatively, McCord (1983) found that parental warmth and affection buffered boys from criminal behavior despite increased risk for criminal involvement due to environmental disadvantages.

Thus, the age-old paradigm of medicine that admonishes the establishment of rapport with the patient holds truth for health behavior change. The three prevention/intervention examples seek to increase bonding, attachment, and connectedness dynamics in varying and differing ways. They all provide an opportunity for parents and youth to become attached. In addition, they all provide educational opportunities for children and their parents. Providing successful educational opportunities creates the "Ah Ha" experience, or the sense of personal mastery. This allows for the development of a strong bond or attachment to the educational service provider, whether they are a parent or school.

In addition, the issue of bonding, attachment, and connectedness dynamics has strong implications for attrition dynamics either in research or service involving non-white populations. Studies reveal that nonwhite populations are difficult to engage in research and treatment (Gorelick, Harris, Burnett, & Bonecutter, 1998; Sue et al., 1995). Thus, all the projects make strenuous attempts not to expose community members to microinsults or to microaggressions (Bell, 1996). We believe that such subtle injuries dissuade poor, nonwhite communities from being attached to the research or the services being offered.

CHAMP

The CHAMP effort to increase bonding, attachment, and connectedness dynamics between parents and their children has essentially involved a strategy of "team learning" (Senge, 1994), or a cooperative learning strategy. Specifically, CHAMP teaches families HIV prevention skills in multiple family groups. CHAMP also teaches family members how to talk and listen to one another. These efforts help Robert Taylor families obtain a sense of person mastery and a clear shared vision (Senge, 1994), that is, the mission to avoid HIV risk behaviors.

CHAMP also provides conveniences to encourage poor, nonwhite community member to become attached to the program either as a CHAMP Collaborative Board member or research subject (Aponte, 1994). Specifically, CHAMP pays its Collaborative Board members and research subjects for their time. Further, board members participate in new "professional" roles at conferences, and obtain jobs as project staff (Madison, McKay, Paikoff & Bell, 2000). In addition, CHAMP board meetings and intervention sessions provide dinner for participants and child care for younger children. The organization holds meetings in an easily accessible Robert Taylor community center, or at their child's school. Community-based staff takes primary responsibility for recruitment and tracking of the sample over time, resulting in high rates of attendance and retention in the program (McCormick et al., 2000). By including community participants in all aspects of CHAMP, we believe this sharply reduces community members' exposure to microinsults and microaggressions; as such community participants are culturally sensitive by definition.

ABAN-AYA

This Afrocentric social development curriculum (SDC) also attempted to increase parental involvement with their children by giving the children various assignments that required parental participation. The aim of these assignments was to provide concrete activities to connect parents and children. In addition, Aban-Aya provided didactic materials that helped children in thinking about their family relations and to strengthen a sense of connectedness with their family and heritage. The Afrocentric SDC curriculum/community development intervention had family/community activities designed to increase the attachment and connectedness dynamics of the participants.

Chicago Board of Education Violence Prevention Initiative

The Chicago Public Schools developed several programs to increase bonding, attachment and connectedness dynamics between parents and CPS and between parents and their children. One program "CPS Parents As Teachers First" called for CPS hiring 600 parents from eighty schools to act as parent-tutor mentors. Their function became to mentor parents to prepare preschoolers for kindergarten by providing developmentally appropriate activities. Thus, preschoolers would obtain academically enriched opportunities, including attention to socially appropriate behavior. Employment opportunities for parents were also provided. This program served more than 2,000 preschoolers during the 1998–1999 school year. "CPS Parents As Teachers First" thus served a dual function—one was to connect parents to CPS, and the other was to help parents connect to their children by helping parents to provide academically enriched opportunities for preschoolers.

CPS's "Cradle to Classroom" provides opportunities for parents to bond with their infants. This long-range prevention strategy allows for infants to grow up with basic trust and security, providing the groundwork for later relationships in life that may prevent violence or intervene in violence. In addition, since pregnancy is the primary reason for high school dropout among urban teens (Dryfoos, 1990; Furstenberg, Brooks-Gunn, & Morgan, 1987), and since many teenage girls with children stop attending school, the "Cradle to Classroom" program allows for teenage mothers to remain in school. By collaborating with Chicago Department of Public Health, six hospitals, and other agencies for pregnant and parenting teens, this program trains teens in the development of parenting skills and accessing community resources. It provides counseling to new mothers around issues of domestic violence and provides teens access to prenatal, nutritional, medical, social, and child care services. This program has significantly reduced dropout rates of teenage mothers in CPS. During the 1998–1999 school year there were 1,100 young women with babies in CPS and 228 of them graduated, with 100 going to college. These young women had only one child despite having the children at very young ages.

CPS has also expanded early childhood services by increasing the number of class-rooms for preschool children so that approximately 25,000 of them, including children with disabilities, are receiving educational services. Thus, more preschool children receive educational services through contractual arrangements with more than forty private and public community-based agencies. By providing quality preschool activities for all children, children have an easier time adapting to the school context and getting attached and connected to school. In addition, these early childhood services allow for the identification of children with attachment disorders by providing 0 to three programs (ZERO TO THREE, 1994) parent/nursing home visitation programs (Olds, Henderson, Chamberlin & Tatelbaum, 1986), and Head Start.

Another strategy the Chicago Public Schools is using to increase the attachment and connectedness dynamics is by expanding the school year. For example, during the summer of 1998, CPS held the largest ever school-based summer programs. Academic programs provide intensive structured instruction for children who do not meet academic promotion standards, for children with significant disabilities, and for children with limited-English-proficiency. In addition, regional competition and camping experiences provide athletic and recreational opportunities. Other efforts, such as the CPS McPrep Lighthouse Program (funded in part by Ronald McDonald Children's Charities), include expanding the school day by providing structured academic activities for children after the regular school day, including a nutritious dinner. These efforts have also served to increase community partnerships with parental involvement. Additionally, all high schools and many elementary schools have competitive and noncompetitive athletic and sports pro-grams after school. In addition, CPS is promoting the use of school uniforms. They require each Local School Council to vote on whether to enact a uniform or dress code policy for the school, and 75% of Chicago public schools have started a uniform or dress code policy.

Efforts are also directed at increasing student attendance and reducing youth drop out rates. Accordingly, CPS has developed a twenty-four hour "Truancy Hot Line" that takes calls from individuals to identify youth who are truant from school to help in truancy pre-vention. CPS truancy prevention services consist of at least two truancy outreach workers at every high school who follow-up on students with unexcused absences. The outreach workers provide counseling services, visit and call youth and parents at home, and daily monitor attendance. Further, regional staff works with all schools to provide assistance in developing programs designed to improve student attendance. There is also a CPS Hispanic dropout prevention program to address the high dropout rate among Hispanic teens. They offer alternative educational and extracurricular activities to all at-risk students of schools where at least 48% percent of the student population is Hispanic.

CPS has developed relationships with alternative schools for youth returning to school. Thirty schools, organized in cooperation with community and social service agen-cies, provide educational services for students who return to school after having dropped out. They provide small class sizes and support services through individual learning plans for each student.

Practitioners seeking to develop an ability to change health behaviors would do well to read Pinderhughes (1979). This work clearly explains the psychophysiology of bonding and attachment behaviors and why they are so important in developing influence over peo-ple. Common sense suggests that trying to teach someone that one lacks a relationship with or has a negative relationship with is a very difficult undertaking. Teaching someone with whom one has a good relationship is much easier.

Self-Esteem

Self-esteem is a feeling that comes from a sense of power, a feeling of being competent to do what must be done, a sense of uniqueness that acknowledges and respects the qualities and characteristics about oneself that are special and different. Self-esteem also means having a sense of models that can be used make sense of the world, and a sense of being connected, a feeling of satisfaction from being connected to people, places or things (Bean, 1992). To change health behavior, improving target recipients' self-esteem is a critical component in any successful prevention/intervention strategy. Bell (1997a) suggests that constructive activities help youth develop social skills and self-esteem that reduce engagement in risky behaviors. All three prevention/intervention examples are firmly grounded in the idea that their efforts needed to improve the self-esteem of their participants.

CHAMP

CHAMP's efforts to improve self-esteem of the recipients started with recognizing that the Robert Taylor residents could collaborate in their own protection from HIV/AIDS. In addition, the strategy of having parents and children engage in team learning by learning skills in multiple family groups has an additional advantage of increasing the participants' self-esteem. In initial work on basic developmental research, feelings of hopelessness and powerlessness in an overwhelming degree surfaced in parents' discussions of risks that concern them regarding their children's health. Such feelings are clearly linked-to self-esteem, and decrease motivation to work on promoting health and preventing risk for one's offspring or themselves. By involving parents directly, first, in helping to delineate stressors and possible areas of influence, and then as key influences over their children's health and well being, we increase self-esteem in at-least two ways. First, parents increase their understanding of their possible influences, and ways they may change their context. Second, parents develop concrete leadership skills, which may help them to further successes in arenas of child rearing, employment, education, and daily living. These effects are likely to be most pronounced for parents who lead CHAMP groups, but potentially affect all parents involved with CHAMP (Madison, McKay, Paikoff & Bell, 2000).

ABAN-AYA

We developed Aban-Aya's activities to increase self-esteem by developing initiatives that give youth a sense of power by teaching them social skills to get them out of high-risk situations. Further, the youth can obtain a sense of models from strategies involved in using the "stop, think, and act" model of decision making (Weissberg, Barton & Shriver, 1997; Weissberg, Jackson & Shriver, 1993). By using African-American values Naguzo Saba (Karenga, 1988) we hoped the African-American children would develop a sense of uniqueness and a sense of being connected. In addition, the SDC/community development condition had activities that would increase the youth's feelings of self-esteem.

Further, the curriculum made it a point to include African-American history, African-American contributions, and African-American proverbs throughout the curriculum to help African-American children develop a sense of power, competence, uniqueness, models, and a sense of being connected, to people, places or things.

Chicago Board of Education Violence Prevention Initiative

One of the Chicago Board of Education's strategies to give youth a sense of power was to incorporate service-learning requirements in the high school curriculum. Another strategy was to improve the academic performance of all students by requiring students, teachers, administrators, and schools to be accountable. Providing learning outcome standards and relevant staff development supported the academic performance of all students. Accordingly, they developed lesson plans consistent with the standards, and made them available to teachers. Establishing a rigorous high school core curriculum, junior and senior high school academies also improved the academic performance of all students, and advisories. Students attending the six regional high schools with academic entrance criteria or the expanded International Baccalaureate programs could also obtain a sense of power. Further, motivated and able students could take college courses by attending local area colleges and universities with which CPS was collaborating. For children having academic difficulty, providing individualized strategies could increase their sense of power. Retained students could improve their deficiencies by tutoring services, smaller class sizes, and specialized curricula.

CPS increases youth's sense of uniqueness of students by providing them the opportunity to find their unique talent. Thus, they can acknowledge and respect the qualities and characteristics about themselves that are special and different. Accordingly, we have provided a wide range of activities for students in the hope that each student can find an area in which his or her unique talents will shine forth.

Character education curricula give youth a sense of models in pre-K through 12th grade by providing educational strategies for strengthening and supporting positive character development. Thus, CPS hopes to help youth in avoiding the high-risk health behavior of violence. In addition, models of conflict resolution are also given. Further, the school curriculum contains information and practice on how youth may avoid or prevent violence by including instruction to reduce racial, ethnic, and religious intolerance. Finally, by giving youth constructive activities that encourage developing skills on how to communicate, solve problems, provide leadership, manage resources, remove barriers to success, and plan, youth will learn models that will help them avoid high risk health behaviors.

Finally, CPS hoped to increase their student's sense of being connected by some previous mentioned strategies found in the increasing bonding, attachment and connectedness dynamics section. In addition, we attempted to increase the feeling of satisfaction from being connected to people, places or things by providing opportunities that encourage attachment to valued people, places, and activities such as mentoring, sports, ROTC, and academic clubs.

Increase Social Skills of Target Recipients

Many researchers (Botvin & Wills, 1985; Cole, 1985; Weissberg & Elias, 1993; Weissberg & Greenberg, 1997) have been longtime proponents of teaching social skills as tools to help youth avoid engaging in risky behaviors. Recognizing this, all three of the prevention/intervention projects sought to increase the social skills of the target recipients that would help in reducing their health risk taking behaviors. In particular, CHAMP and Aban-Aya have been interested in improving youth's assertiveness and refusal skills, and their understanding of potentially risky situations. In other words, CHAMP and Aban-Aya

(SDC/community condition) attempt to prepare youth for dealing with risky contexts, while simultaneously hoping to improve these contexts (making them less risky).

CHAMP

In helping youth avoid contracting HIV/AIDS, CHAMP teaches youth sexual behavior refusal skills. In addition, CHAMP teaches youth safer sex skills, so that if youth do become sexually active, they are better prepared. Research has shown programming that stresses abstinence—but providing "just in case" information regarding safer sex—is highly effective for a wide range of urban youth (Jemmott and Jemmott, 1998). In line with Elliott and Tolan (1999), who note "successful family interventions have combined behavioral parent training techniques with other intervention components based in family systems theory that are designed to improve family relations," CHAMP works to help youth develop good communication skills by helping youth and parents learn about and practice their communication skills in multiple family groups. We also give parents social skills that help them in supervision and monitoring of the child and increase involvement with the child as well as knowledge of children's activities and whereabouts. We also teach parents the social skills that involve the use of positive parenting.

ABAN-AYA

Aban-Aya's Afrocentric risk behavior prevention curriculum teaches skills to refuse offers and resist social pressure, assertiveness, negotiation and conflict resolution, and gives youth the opportunity to practice these skills to aid in their ability to avoid high risk health behaviors. These social skills are taught in the context of learning decision making ("Stop, Think and Act") and problem solving skills. Understanding the feelings of self and others (empathy), goal setting, and other self-management skills are also taught.

Chicago Board of Education Violence Prevention Initiative

CPS's efforts to increase the social skills of its target recipients include providing educational opportunities for infants, toddlers, and preschoolers, and their parents. This strategy creates the opportunity to develop life skills and social skills necessary to prevent and intervene in violence. By giving youth opportunities to serve their community, resolve disputes peacefully and develop leadership skills that will enable them to model and promote healthy alternatives to violence, CPS hopes to give youth social skills to help in avoiding the high-risk health behavior of violence. Thus, schools are providing opportunities to be involved with a Teen Court program. In addition, in the CPS Peer Leaders Program, elementary and high school leaders teach students peer mediation, conflict resolution, and anger management skills. Further, the CPS Young Negotiators program teaches student negotiation skill. In the CPS Peer Mediation program students learn from peers to manage conflict and disagreements using a diversity of techniques. Such techniques allow them to avoid violence and other forms of aggressive and antisocial behavior. Finally, by being involved in mentoring programs and service clubs, youth learn additional social skills.

CPS is also providing support to school staff and parents to improve their ability to teach children appropriate social skills and to use positive interventions to decrease disruptive student behavior. Thus, CPS School Climate Teams help in the development of safety plans that schools include in their School Improvement Plans. School Climate Teams cooperate with Crisis Intervention teams, Interfaith, and School and Community Relations staff to help in school crises situations. The CPS Boys' Town Educational Model provides a social/life skill's curriculum training model that provides intervention strategies to school personnel. The CPS Behavior Management Training program provides training upon request from schools, teachers, and educational support staff. It teaches team techniques to modify students' disruptive and aggressive behavior and helps students develop control and socially proactive behavior. School personnel in twenty schools receive training on how to help in diffusing volatile behavior and teach students proactive behavior. School personnel in twenty schools receive training on how to help in diffusing volatile behavior and teach students proactive behavior. Finally, the CPS Behavior Intervention Teachers are specialists who provide proactive assistance to teachers who need to enhance their behavior management skills to deal with violent and hostile behavior. They help school personnel in developing individual behavior management plans for students.

Reestablishing the Adult Protective Shield

Pynoos and Nader (1988) discuss reestablishing the adult protective shield as a psychological first aid measure to deal with the child's generalized anxiety when confronted with a traumatic stressor. The authors believe that this concept is also extremely useful in helping individuals to make health behavior changes. As previously pointed out, communities with social fabric clearly have less "deviant behavior." This is due to the prevention of promulgation of this deviant behavior (Sampson et al., 1997), and this may depend on reestablishing the adult protective shield. The social disorganization theory of deviance, which attributes the deterioration of community social fabric as causing reduced informal and formal social control (Shaw & McKay, 1942), can be interpreted as a deterioration of the adult protective shield. As evidenced in all three prevention/intervention projects, this reestablishment of the adult protective shield is considered a key component in the health behavior change efforts.

CHAMP

As has been mentioned earlier, a key component of CHAMP has been the issue of ameliorating contexts for children. CHAMP sees families as key to ameliorating contexts, and attempts to help families in many ways. First, if we monitor children intensively, contexts by default are less risky. CHAMP works with parents to stress the importance of monitoring from the perspective of keeping kids out of risky situations. CHAMP also works with kids to underscore the reasons parents must monitor their children. However, monitoring children in an urban setting is fraught with problems, and requires substantial family support. Therefore, CHAMP stresses both internal and external support systems, hoping to link families together through multiple family groups and thus to increase potential monitoring resources. Such changes ideally result in a neighborhood "village" where the adult protective shield consists of many in the community, all of whom we can trust to look out for the welfare of the child.

ABAN-AYA

Increasing family involvement with children is also a central concern in Aban-Aya. Materials are sent home to parents informing them of the importance of communicating with their children and ways of doing that. Many homework activities require the child to engage and communicate with their parents. In the SDC curriculum/community condition, parents are also offered Parent Education Workshops where they learn how to improve their parenting skills and attachment with their children.

Chicago Board of Education Violence Prevention Initiative

By strictly enforcing disciplinary rules while providing a safety net of school-based educational opportunities for expelled youth, youth who have violated probation, or have committed first time, but nonviolent, serious offenses, CPS reestablishes the adult protective shield. The CPS Zero Tolerance/Alternative Programs contain a Uniform Discipline Code that established consequences for student misconduct. Students found to posses illegal drugs, firearms, or other dangerous weapons have immediate consequences, including expulsion and referral to an alternative school. Fortunately, there are six alternative school sites available for 500 students expelled from school, or referred for chronically disruptive behavior, that allows for continual monitoring of these problematic youth. These schools have small class sizes and provide support services through individual learning plans for each student.

In addition, CPS has a Saturday Morning Alternative Reach Out and Teach Program (SMART). In this program, first time drug or alcohol offenders get taught a curriculum that focuses on character education, leadership development, conflict resolution training, gang prevention and detachment, and substance abuse counseling. Students meet on seven consecutive Saturdays, including two with their parents. Further, CPS expects each student to provide twenty hours of community service and they give each a mentor. They refer students who do not successfully complete the program for expulsion. In collaboration with the Cook County Probation Department, CPS Operation Jump Start gives intensive support to youth who are under the jurisdiction of the probation department. Jump Start also provides youth who have had significant educational problems extensive instruction in social skills and back-to-school transitional support. Following the eight-week program, youth attend either an alternative or regular school.

The Chicago Public Schools are also reestablishing the adult protective shield by implementing safety and security programs designed to maximize school safety. CPS has developed parent patrols that exist in more than 200 schools. In this initiative, parents patrol the streets before and after school to ensure safe travel. They train parents in safety and security measures, and participate in workshops on safety, violence, and conflict resolution. CPS has also enhanced training and expansion of security personnel by assigning more than 600 professional security personnel to CPS schools. Further, CPS, with the Chicago Police Department, provides two-person teams of uniformed police officers who work eight-hour shifts at each high school. The Chicago Police Department and the Office of Specialized Services provide monthly training to enable them to work proactively with students and the school community. Targeted training includes cultural awareness, diversity and sensitivity, internal and external school linkages, positive intervention techniques, de-escalating aggressive behavior, referral procedures and resources, and communication skills. There is also assistance for schools in the development of individualized school security programs.

CPS also began Operation S.A.F.E. (Schools Are For Education). This is a system of rapid response teams consisting of officers in a mobile tactical unit. These teams patrol the vicinity immediately surrounding high schools and can respond quickly to any emergency calls. A rapid response team, composed of part-time police officers, supplements the high school mobile tactical unit. Part-time officers who patrol the city after hours respond to alarms and break-ins at schools, and form the CPS Night Stalkers program. These efforts help to reduce burglaries, vandalism, and theft after school hours. They also give informational booklets to parents on the safe passage of students to and from school. The CPS Safe Passage booklet provided to principals and parents, offer helpful tips to keep children safe on their way to and from school, and in their neighborhoods during non-school hours. They provide parents and students tips including the use of the buddy system, following a designated safety route, and designating safe havens within the community.

Finally, there are metal detectors in every middle and high school. They install metal detectors in 90% of the system's high schools and a few elementary schools. These have been responsible for recovering many weapons that may otherwise have gone undetected. Paul Vallas C.E.O. of the schools notes that CPS metal detectors detected 100 guns in 1997. Such efforts create awareness between students and community that the adult protective shield is in existence and it will not tolerate weapons and illegal contraband.

One of the initiatives CPS began to increase the monitoring behavior of parents of children in Chicago Public Schools was to require parents to pick up their youth's report cards during a "parent report card pick up day." They designed this activity to allow parents and teachers an opportunity to collaborate on monitoring the student's academic performance and classroom behavior. In addition, ninety percent of CPS high schools have security cameras or complete surveillance systems, which monitor hallways, stairwells, remote areas, and the perimeter of the campuses. These endeavors have significantly reduced vandalism. Also, the Chicago Board of Education provides monitoring of youth by providing truancy services, increasing summer school, and enriching school activities.

In summary, family communication, school-wide climate changes, and community connections can be risk or protective factors which lead to increased or decreased negative outcomes. Protective approaches improve children's attachment/bonding to positive family, school, community values and beliefs, and lessen the chances of maladaptive outcomes in the presence of risks (Garbarino, 1993; Garmezy, 1993; Grossman et al., 1992; Rutter, 1987; Masten et al., 1990). Effective programs must increase protective factors for students, by increasing their involvement with communal institutions of family, school and peers. Family-oriented intervention to change parenting style and practices can reduce risk or serious antisocial behavior and violence by increasing predictability, parental monitoring of children and decreasing negative parenting methods. Lack of parental monitoring, represented at its extreme by neglect and poor discipline methods and conflict about discipline, has been related to participation in delinquent and violent behavior for a range of populations (Farrington, 1989; Gorman-Smith et al., 1996; Patterson, 1992).

Minimizing Effects of Trauma

Behind all anger is hurt and attached to the hurt is fear of being hurt again. Unfortunately, such emotions often cause individuals to engage in health risk taking behaviors involving anger, sex and drug use. Thus, to help individuals change their health behaviors, we need to address the issue of traumatic stress that causes the original hurt. Accordingly, we must develop a level of sensitivity to identify trauma in children (Bell & Jenkins, 1993). There needs to be provision of crisis intervention teams to address traumatic stress (Allen et al., 1999). Further, the effects of subtle long-term trauma need to be addressed with therapy (Pynoos & Nader, 1988). A major strategy of addressing issues of traumatic stress is to transform traumatic helplessness into learned helpfulness (Appel & Simon, 1996).

CHAMP and ABAN-AYA

Although CHAMP and Aban-Aya recognize the importance of this issue, due to the limited scope of the research we did not include this in the intervention. It is done on an informal manner. In CHAMP, all intervention groups have trained mental health interns who have been particularly sensitive to these issues, given the nature of the program. Thus, when stress related problems surface, CHAMP staff have sought out treatment services and made problems surface, CHAMP staff have sought out treatment services and made referrals. Aban-Aya staff has made similar interventions when they have identified similar problems.

Chicago Board of Education Violence Prevention Initiative

The mental health professionals at the Chicago Public School have long observed the impact of traumatic stress on the youth they serve (Dyson, 1990). Accordingly, the CPS Specialized Services developed the CPS Crisis Intervention Services program that provides pupil support teams. In addition, the Interfaith Partnerships and community-based social and health services supplement these services. These services provide prevention, intervention, and post-vention counseling activities to reduce the possibility and impact of violent acts. The Chicago Public School Specialized Services Department requires all schools have at least one counselor who can help students who are having difficulty in school or at home and a team that includes a nurse, psychologist, and social worker. Individual and small group counseling are part of the school pupil support services program. However, whenever the students' needs are beyond the school's resources, they refer the student to other programs or agencies. To turn learned helplessness into learned helpfulness, the Chicago Public Schools have developed community service demands for students. As a required component of the high school curriculum, students will provide a minimum of forty hours in service learning. They must engage in such activities as tutoring, working with elders, community beautification projects, etc. Teens will show their learning through presentations, papers, portfolios, etc.

Summary

This chapter covers the seven basic field principles necessary to effect health behavior changes in large populations. These principles—(1) rebuilding the village, (2) providing access to health care, (3) improving bonding, attachment, and connectedness dynamics within the community and between stakeholders, (4) improving self-esteem, (5) increasing social skills of target recipients, (6) reestablishing the adult protective shield and monitoring and (7) minimizing the residual effects of trauma—are based on academic theoretical constructs which have been modified to inform field work. The authors have illustrated these seven principles by using three examples, two research projects and on naturalistic study, that highlight the principles.

References

Ainsworth, M.D.S. (1973). The development of infant-mother attachment. In B. M. Caldwell & H.N. Ricciuti (Eds.), *Review of child development research*: Vol. 3 (pp. 1–95). Chicago: University of Chicago Press.

Ajzen I. (1985). From decisions to actions: A theory of planned behavior. In J. Kuhl & J. Beckmann (Eds.), *Action-control: From cognition to behavior* (Pp. 11–39). Heidelberg: Springer.

Akers, R.L., Krohn, M.D., Lanza-Kaduce, L., & Radosevich, M. (1979). Social learning and deviant behavior: A specific test of a general theory. *American Sociological Review*, 44, 636–655.

Allen, S.F., Dlugokinski, E.L., Cohen, L.A., & Walker, J.L. (1999). Assessing the impact of a traumatic community event on children and assisting their healing. *Psychiatric Annals*, 29(2), 93–98.

American Psychiatric Association (1994). *Diagnostic and Statistical Manual*—Fourth Edition. Washington, D.C.: American Psychiatric Press.

American Psychiatric Association (1996). Practice guideline for the treatment of patients with nicotine dependence. Supplement to the *American Journal Of Psychiatry*, 153 (10).

Apfel, R.J & Simon, B. (Eds.) (1996). *Minefields in their hearts* (Pp. 9–11).—New Haven: Yale University Press.

Aponte, J.F., Young-Rivers, R., & Wohl, J. (Eds.) (1995). *Psychological Interventions and Cultural Diversity*. Boston: Allyn & Bacon.

Aponte, H. (1994). Bread and spirit: Therapy with the new poor. New York: W.W. Norton.

Baker, F.M. & Bell, C.C. (1999). African Americans: Treatment concerns. *Psychiatric Services*, 50(3), 362–368.

Bandura, A. (1977). *Social learning theory*. Englewood Cliffs, NJ: Prentice-Hall.

Bandura, A. (1986). *Social foundations of thought and action*. Englewood Cliffs, NJ: Prentice-Hall.

Bean, R. (1992). *The four conditions of self-esteem: A new approach for elementary and middle schools*, Ed 2. Santa Cruz, CA: ETR Associates.

Bell, C.C. (1997a). Promotion of mental health through coaching of competitive sports. *Journal of the National Medical Association*, 89(8), 517–520.

Bell, C.C. (1997b). Taking issue: Doesn't anyone remember the dangers of lead? *Psychiatric Services*. 48(3), 273.

Bell, C.C. & Jenkins, E.J. (1993). Community violence and children on Chicago's Southside. *Psychiatry: Interpersonal and Biological Processes*, 56(1), 46–54.

Bell, C.C., Gamm, S., Vallas, P. & Jackson, P. (2001). Strategies for the prevention of youth violence in Chicago public schools. In M. Shafii & S. Shafii (Eds.). *School violence: Contributing factors, management, and prevention* (pp 251–272). Washington, D.C.: American Psychiatric Press.

Bowlby, J. (1973). *Attachment and loss:* Vol. 2. Separation. New York: Basic Books.

Booth, C.L., Spieker, S.J., Barnard, K.E., & Morisset, C.E. (1992). Infants at risk: The role of preventive intervention in deflecting a maladaptive developmental trajectory. In J. McCord and R.E. Tremblay (Eds.), *Preventing antisocial behavior: Interventions from birth through adolescence* (Pp. 21–42). New York: Guilford Press.

Borduin, C., Cone, L., Mann, B. et al. (1985). *Changed lives: The effects of the Perry School Preschool on youths through age 19*. Ypsilanti, MI: High Scope Press.

Botvin, G.J. & Wills, T.A. (1985). Personal and social skills training: Cognitive-behavioral approaches to substance abuse prevention. In P. Bell & R. Battjes, (Eds.), *Prevention research: Deterring drug abuse among children and adolescents*. (Series #63, Pp. 67–112) Washington, D.C.: NIDA Research Monograph.

Bronfenbrenner, U. (1979). *The ecology of human development*. London: Cambridge University Press.

Coie, J.D. (1985). Fitting social skills intervention to the target group. In B. Schneider, K. Rubin & J.E. Ledingham (Eds.) *Children's peer relations: Issues in assessment and intervention* (Pp. 141–156). New York: Springer-Verlag.

Comer, J.P. (1988). Educating poor minority children. *Scientific American*. 259 (5), 42–48.

Digman, J.M. (1990). Personality structure: Emergence of the five-factor model. *Ann Rev of Psychology*, 41, 417–440.

Dryfoos, J.G. (1990). Prevalence of adolescent pregnancy. *In Adolescents at risk: Prevalence and Prevention* (Pp. 72–73). New York: Oxford University Press.

Dyson, J.L. (1980). The effect of family violence on children's academic performance and behavior. *Journal of The National Medical Association*, 82 (1), 17–22.

Earls, F. (1991). A developmental approach to understanding and controlling violence. In H.E. Fitzgerald (Ed.) *Theory and research in behavioral pediatrics*, Vol. 4 (Pp. 61–88). New York: Plenum Press.

Elliot, D.S., Huizinga, D. & Ageton, S.S. (1985). *Explaining delinquency and drug use*. Beverly Hills: Sage.

Elliott, D.S. & Tolan, P.H. (1999). Youth violence prevention, intervention, and social policy: An Overview. In D.J. Flannery & C.R. Huff (Eds.) Youth violence: prevention, intervention and social policy (Pp. 3–46). Washington, D.C.: American Psychiatric Press.

Eron, L. D., Huesmann, L.R. & Zelli, A. (1991). The role of parental variables in the learning of aggression. In D. Pepler & K. Rubin (Eds.) *The development and treatment of childhood aggression* (Pp. 171–188). Hillsdale, NJ: Erlbaum.

Farrington, D.P. (1989). Early predictors of adolescent aggression and adult violence. *Violence and Victims*, 4, 79–100.

Fishbein, M. & Ajzen, I. (1975). *Belief, attitude, intention and behavior: An Introduction theory and research*. Reading, MA: Addison-Wesley.

Flay, B.R. & Petraitis, J. (1994). The theory of triadic influence: A new theory of health behavior with implications for preventive interventions. In G.S. Albrecht (Ed.) *Advances In Medical Sociology*, Vol. IV: A Reconsideration of Models of Health Behavior Change (Pp. 19–44). Greenwich, CT: JAI Press.

Flay, B.R. et al. (In Progress). *The Aban-Aya Youth Project*. University of Illinois at Chicago.

Furstenberg, F.F., Brooks-Gunn, J. & Morgan, S.P. (1987). *Adolescent mothers in later life*. New York: Cambridge University Press.

Garbarino, J. (1993), Children's response to community violence: What do we know? *Infant Mental Health Journal*, 14, 103–115.

Garmezy, N. (1993). Children in poverty: Resilience Despite Risk. *Psychiatry: interpersonal and biological processes*, 56, 127–136.

Gorelick, P.B., Harris, Y., Bumett, B., & Bonecutter, F.J. (1998). The recruitment triangle: Reasons why African Americans enroll, refuse to enroll, or voluntarily withdraw from a clinical trial. *Journal of The National Medical Association*, 90, 141–145.

Gorman-Smith, D. et al. (1996). The relation of family functioning to violence among inner-city minority youths. *Journal of Family Psychology*, 10, 115–129.

Grossman, F.K., Beinashowitz, J., Anderson, L., Sakurai, M., Finnin, L. & Flaherty, M. (1992). Risk and resilience in young adolescents. *Journal of Youth and Adolescence*, 21, 529–549.

Guerra, N. (1997). Intervening to prevent childhood aggression in the inner city. In J. McCord (Ed.) *Violence and childhood in the inner city*. (Pp. 256–312). Cambridge, UK: Cambridge University Press.

Hatch, J., Moss, N., Saran, A., Presley-Cantrell, L., Mallory, C. (1993). Community research: Partnership in Black Communities. *American Journal of Preventive Medicine*, 9 (6, Suppl), 27–31.

Haynes, N.M. & Comer, J.P. (1996). Integrating schools, families, and communities through successful school reform: The school development program. *School Psychology Review*, 25(4), 501–506.

Haynes, N.M., Comer, J.P. & Hamilton-Lee, M. (1989). School climate enhancement through parental involvement. *Journal of School Psychology*, 27, 87–90.

Henggeler, S.W., Melton, G.B., & Smith, L.A. (1992). Family preservation using multi-systemic therapy: An effective alternative to incarcerating serious juvenile offenders. *Journal of Consulting Clinical Psychology*, 60, 953–961.

Howard, M. & McCabe, J.A. (1992). An information and skills approach for younger teens. In B.C. Miller, J.J. Card, R.L. Paikoff, & J.L. Peterson (Eds.) *Preventing adolescent pregnancy* (Pp. 83–109). Newbury Park: CA: Sage.

Jemmott, J.B., Jemmott, L.S., & Fong, G.T. (1998). Abstinence and safer sex HIV risk-reduction interventions for African American adolescents: A randomized controlled trial. *Journal of the American Medical Association*, 279, 19, 1529–1536.

Jemmott, J.B., Jemmott, L.S. & Fong, G.T. (1992). Reductions in HIV risk-associated sexual behaviors among Black male adolescents: Effects of an AIDS prevention intervention. *American Journal of Public Health*, 82, 372–377.

Karenga, M. (1988). *The African American holiday of Kwanzaa: A celebration of family, community & culture*. Los Angeles: University of Sankore Press.

Klein, R.G., Abikoff, H., Klass, E., Ganeles, D., Seese, L.M., & Pollack, S. (1997). Clinical efficacy of methylphenidate in conduct disorder with and without attention deficit Hyperactivity Disorder. *Archives of General Psychiatry*, 54, 1073–1080.

Lewis, D.O., Moy, E., Jackson, L.D. et al. (1985). Biosocial characteristics of children who later murder: A prospective study. *American Journal of Psychiatry*, 142, 1161–1167.

Madison, S., McKay, M.M., Paikoff, R., Bell, C.C. (2000). Basic research and community collaboration: necessary ingredients for the development of a Family-based HIV prevention Program. *AIDS Education and Prevention*, 12(4), 281–298.

Masten, A.S., Best, K.M., & Garmezy, N. (1990). Resilience and development: Contributions from the study of children who overcome adversity. *Development and Psychopathology*, 2, 425–444.

McBride, C. & Paikoff, R. (1999). Family influences on the onset of sexual activity among adolescents. Presented at the NIMH Families and AIDS Conference, Philadelphia, Pennsylvania.

McCord, J. (1983). A forty-year perspective on the effects of child abuse and neglect. *Child Abuse and Neglect*, 7, 265–270.

McCormick, A. M., McKay, M.M., Wilson, M., McKinney, L., Paikoff, R., Bell, C., Baptiste, D., Coleman, D, Gillming, G., Madison, S., & Scott, R. (2000). Involving families in an urban HIV prevention intervention: How community collaboration addresses barriers to participation. *AIDS Education and Prevention*, 12(4), 299–307.

McKay, M.M., Baptiste, D. Coleman, D., Madison, S., Paikaff, R., & Scott, R. (2000). Preventing HIV risk exposure in urban communities: The CHAMP family program. Pequenot, W. & Szapocznik (Eds.) (pp. 67–87). Thousand Oaks, CA: Sage.

Meloy, R. (1992). *Violent attachments*. New Jersey: Jason Aronson, Inc.

Miller, B.C., Card, J.J., Paikoff, R.L., & Peterson, J.L. (1992). *Preventing adolescent pregnancy*. Newbury Park, CA: Sage.

Moffitt, T.E. (1997). Neuropsychology, antisocial behavior, and neighborhood context. In J. McCord (Ed.). *Violence and childhood in the inner city* (Pp. 116–170). Cambridge UK: Cambridge University Press.

Olds, D.L., Henderson, C.R., Chamberlin, R., & Tatelbaum, R. (1986). Preventing child abuse and neglect: A randomized trial of nurse home visitation. *Pediatrics*, 78, 65–78.

Oetting, E.R. & Beauvais, R. (1986). Peer cluster theory: Drugs and the adolescent. *Journal of Counseling and Development*, 65, 17–22.

Oetting, E.R. & Beauvais, F. (1990–91). Orthogonal cultural identification theory: The cultural identification of minority adolescents. *International Journal of the Addictions*, 25, (5A & 6A), 655–685.

Paikoff, R.L. (1997). Applying developmental psychology to an AIDS prevention model for urban African-American youth. *Journal of Negro Education*, 65, 44–59.

Paikoff, R.L. (1995). Early heterosexual debut: Situations of sexual possibility. *American Journal of Orthopsychiatry*, 65(3), 389–401.

Paikoff, R.L., McBride, C., McCormick, A., McKay, M., McKinney, L. & McCormick, S. (In Progress). Interviewing pre and young adolescents about heterosocial and heterosexual experiences: Longitudinal and cross-sample comparisons. *The CHAMP Project*, University of Illinois at Chicago.

Petraitis, J., Flay, B.R., & Miller, T.Q. (1995). Reviewing theories of adolescent substance abuse: Organizing pieces of the puzzle. *Psychological Bulletin*, 117(1), 67–86.

Pinderhughes, C.A. (1979). Differential bonding: Toward a psychophysiological theory of stereotyping. *American Journal of Psychiatry*, 136, 33–37.

Pinderhughes, C.A. (1972). Managing paranoia in violent relationships. In G. Usdin (Ed.) *Perspectives on Violence* (Pp. 111–139). New York: Brunner/Mazel.

Pynoos, R. & Nader, K. (1988). Psychological first aid for children who witness community violence. *Journal of Traumatic Stress*, 1(4), 445–473.

Renken, B., Egeland, B., Marvinney, D., Mangelsdorf, S., & Sroufe, L.A. (1989). Early childhood antecedents of aggression and passive-withdrawal in early elementary school. *Journal of Personality*, 57, 257–281.

Resnick, M.D., Bearman, P.S., Blum, R.W., et al. (1997). Protecting adolescents from harm: Findings from the National Longitudinal Study on Adolescent Health. *Journal of the American Medical Association*, 278(10), 823–832.

Rutter, M. (1987). Psychosocial resilience and protective mechanisms. *American Journal of Orthopsychiatry*, 57, 316–331.

Sampson, R.J., Raudenbush, S.W., & Earls, F. (1997). Neighborhoods and violent crime: A Multilevel Study of Collective Efficacy. *Science*, 277, 918–924.

Senge, P. (1994). *The Fifth Discipline*. New York: Doubleday.

Shaw, C.R. & McKay, H. (1942). *Juvenile delinquency and urban areas*. Chicago: University of Chicago Press.

Smith, P., Flay, B.R., Bell, C.C., & Weissberg, R.P. (2001). The protective influence of parents and peers in violence avoidance among African-American youth. *Maternal and Child Health Journal*, 5(4), 245–252.

Sroufe, L.A., Egeland, B., Kreutzer, T. (1990). The fate of early experience following developmental change: Longitudinal approaches to individual adaptation in childhood. *Child Development*, 61(5), 1363–1373.

Sue, S., Chun, C. & Gee, K. (1995), Ethnic minority intervention and research. In J.F. Aponte, R. Young-Rivers, & J. Wohl (Eds.) *Psychological interventions and cultural diversity* (pp. 266–282). Boston: Allyn & Bacon.

Szapocznik, J. (1996). Family and cultural processes in primary and secondary prevention. Presentation made at the IX international conference on HIV/AIDS, July 1996, Vancouver, British Columbia, Canada.

Tolan, P.H. & Lorion, R.P. (1988). Multivariate approaches to the identification of delinquency—proneness in males. *American Journal of Community Psychology*, 16, 547–561.

Tolan, P.H. & McKay, M.M. (1996). Preventing aggression in urban children: An empirically based family prevention program. *Family Relations*, 45: 148–155.

Tolan, P.H., Mitchell, M.E. (1989). Families and the therapy of antisocial delinquent behavior. *Journal of Psychotherapy and The Family*, 6, 29–48.

Weissberg, R.P., Barton, H.A., & Shriver, T.P. (1997). The social-competence promotion program for young adolescents. In G.W. Albee & T.P. Gullotta (Eds.), *Primary prevention exemplars: the Lela Rowland awards* (Pp. 268–290). Thousand Oaks, CA: Sage.

Weissberg, R.P. & Elias, M.J. (1993). Enhancing young people's social competence and health behavior. *Applied and Preventive Psychology*, 3, 179–190.

Weissberg, R.P. & Greenberg, T. (1997). School and community competence enhancement and prevention programs. In E. Sigel & K.A. Renninger (Eds.). *Handbook Of Child Psychology:* Vol. 4—Child psychology in practice (5th Ed). New York: John Wiley.

Weissberg, R.P., Jackson, A.S. & Shriver, T.P. (1993). Promoting positive social development and health practices in young urban adolescents. In M.J. Elias (Ed.) *Social decision-making and life skills development: guidelines for middle school educators* (Pp. 45–77). Gaithersburg, MD: Aspen Publications.

Zero to three. (1994). *Caring for infants and toddlers in violent environments:* Hurt, healing, and hope. Washington, D.C.

Chapter **3**

Cultural Competence in Behavioral Health Care

DERALD WING SUE

In addition to the normal health problems encountered in life, racial/ethnic minorities are often subjected to the stressors of minority status in our society. A large body of literature exists indicating that racism is a continuing stressor in the lives of persons of color; that they are subjected to prejudice, bias and discrimination, education, housing, and employment; and that they are more likely to live in poverty (Jones, 1997; President's Initiative on Race, 1998; D.W. Sue & Sue, 1999; Clark, Anderson, Clark, & Williams, 1999).

The detrimental consequences of racism on the physical and psychological well being of racial/ethnic minorities are well documented. For example, the health status for persons of color reveals disturbing disparities related to life span, death rates, and susceptibility to illnesses; African American life expectancy in 1990 was 69.1 years compared to 76.1 for Whites (Jones, 1998); excess death rates for blacks under 70 were 42.3%, for American Indians 25%, and for Hispanics 14% (Williams, Lavizzo-Mourey, & Warren, 1994). There are generally higher rates of infant mortality and homicide among persons of color; poorer diets were characteristic of many minority groups; and they were more likely to be prone to diseases, diabetes, and hypertension (U.S. Department of Health and Human Services, 1985; Williams and Collins, 1995). In the area of mental health, it has been found that racism affects the psychological well being of African Americans, Asian Americans, Latino Americans and Native Americans (Parham, Whit, & Ajamu, 1999; D.W. Sue & Sue, 1999; Herring, 1997).

While it would appear that adequate health care for minorities is a pressing necessity, the nature of medical services for racial/ethnic minority populations is woefully inadequate and biased (Jones, 1997; Presidents Initiative on Race, 1998; Hall, 1999). A higher proportion of minorities and people of color are medically uninsured, are less likely to be insured by Medicaid, and/or live in medically underserved areas. Even when given access to medical care, that care is often inadequate, inferior and more likely to result in the death of racial/ethnic minority patients. In one large-scale nationwide study of 11,000 patients, for example, researchers at Memorial Sloan-Kettering Cancer Center in New York found: (1) African Americans are more likely to receive substandard treatment; (2) if Black patients would have been given identical medical treatment as their White counterparts, they would have increased their survival rate by 308%; and (3) evidence is strong that bias on the part of physicians influence access to optimal cancer cures (Hall, 1999).

In light of the increasing diversity of our society, health care professionals inevitably will be encountering patient populations, which differ from them in terms of race, culture, and ethnicity. Yet, the theories of health care, the standards used to judge healthy and unhealthy behavior, and the actual delivery of services are culture-bound and reflect a monocultural perspective of the health care professions. As such, the practice of public health is often culturally inappropriate and antagonistic to the lifestyles and values of minority groups in our society. As an example, some professionals of color assert that the helping professions are "handmaidens of the status quo", "instruments of oppression" and "transmitters of society's values" (D.W. Sue, Carter et al., 1999; Carter, 1995). The presence of structural inequities in the delivery of services, intentional and unintentional discrimination by providers, and the limited cultural competency of providers are at the root of these allegations (President's Initiative on Race, 1998).

Ethnocentric Monoculturalism

The health care professions are culturally encapsulated at the individual, professional, organizational and societal levels. As such, our communities of color have definitions of illness and treatment imposed upon them. Fighting the profession's biased assumptions and structural inequities means a struggle against the ethnocentric monoculturalism at the core of our inability to deal effectively with matters of health behavior influenced by race, culture, ethnicity, gender and sexual orientation. The dynamics of ethnocentric monoculturalism are listed below (D.W. Sue & Sue, 1999).

First, there is a strong belief in the superiority of one group's cultural heritage (history, values, language, traditions, arts/crafts, etc.). White/Euro American norms and values are seen positively, and descriptors may include such terms as "more advanced" and "more civilized." Members of the society and the health care professions may possess conscious and unconscious feelings of superiority, and feel that their way of doing things is the "best way". Western science, which guides health care practice, is considered to be a "superior form of treatment." Indigenous forms of treatment are considered "inferior and unscientific." Such an ethnocentric practice may clash with many Eastern beliefs about good medical intervention. Many Asian Americans and Pacific Islanders, for example, prefer alternative practitioners such as herbalists, acupuncturists or chi gung specialists. Because they are not considered mainstream forms of treatment, reimbursements by insurance carriers for these therapies may be denied.

Second, there is a belief in the inferiority of all other groups' cultural heritage, which extends to their customs, values, traditions and language. Other societies, communities of color, or groups may be perceived as "less developed," "uncivilized, "primitive" or even "pathological." The lifestyle or ways of doing things by the group are considered inferior as evidenced by the example above. The mental health professions, for example, often act as if other societies never had anything like counseling and psychotherapy until Euro Americans invented it.

Third, the dominant group possesses the power to impose their standards and beliefs upon the less powerful group. This component of ethnocentric monoculturalism is very important. All groups are to some extent ethnocentric; that is, they feel positive about their cultural heritage and way of life. Yet, if they do not possess the power to impose their values on others, they hypothetically cannot oppress. It is power or the unequal status relationship between groups that defines ethnocentric monoculturalism.

Fourth, the ethnocentric values and beliefs are manifested in the programs, policies, practices, structures and institutions of the society. For example, chain-of-command systems, training and educational systems, communication systems, management systems, performance appraisal systems and conventional health care delivery systems often dictate and control our lives. They attain untouchable and godfather-like status in an organization and profession. Because most systems are monocultural in nature and demand compliance, racial/ethnic minorities may be oppressed.

Five, since service providers are all products of cultural conditioning, their values and beliefs (worldview) represent an invisible veil, which operates outside the level of conscious awareness. As a result, health care providers may assume universality; that everyone regardless of race, culture, ethnicity or gender shares the nature of reality and truth. This assumption is erroneous, but seldom questioned because it is firmly ingrained in our worldview.

Overcoming ethnocentric monoculturalism is one of the major barriers to becoming culturally competent at the individual, professional, organizational and societal levels. Providers often do not understand the ways that cultural influences affect them and their patients as they deliver medical services. They fail to be aware and respectful of their patients' cultural values and beliefs, and allow racial stereotyping and language barriers to result in denied or delayed treatment. The cultural competency gap is even more disturbing when one realizes that the medical establishment is disproportionately White and becoming more so (President's Initiative on Race, 1998). For example the percentage of first-year medical students who are African American, Latino American or Native American is dropping, while the percentage of their population is growing.

Cultural Competence of Health Care Providers

Achieving cultural competence means the following (D.W. Sue, Arredondo, & McDavis, 1992; D.W. Sue, Carter et al., 1998):

1. Health care professionals must all become culturally aware of their own values, biases, and assumptions about human behavior.

- What stereotypes, perceptions and beliefs do they hold about culturally different groups and communities, which may hinder their ability to form a helpful and effective relationship with individual clients, client groups and minority constituents?
- What are the worldviews they bring to the clinical encounter?
- What value systems are inherent in their theory of health care, and what values underlie the nature and manner in their provision of services?

Without such an awareness and understanding, health care providers may inadvertently assume that everyone, shares their worldview. When this happens, the health care professional may become guilty of cultural oppression, imposing values on their culturally different clients and communities.

2. The health care professional must acquire knowledge and understanding of the worldview of minority or culturally different groups and clients.

- What biases, values and assumptions about human behavior do these groups hold?
- Is there such a thing as an African American, Asian American, Latino (a)/Hispanic American or American Indian worldview?
- How might this affect assessment/therapeutic processes and goals?

Knowledge of the history, life experiences, cultural values, and the hopes, fears and aspirations of culturally different groups in the United States is crucial to becoming a culturally competent provider.

3. Health care professionals must begin the process of developing culturally appropriate and effective health care interventions in working with culturally different clients and communities. This means prevention as well as remediation approaches, and systems intervention as well as traditional one-to-one relationships. Equally important is the ability to make use of existing indigenous-helping/healing approaches, which may already exist in the minority community.

4. Health care professionals must begin to understand how organizational and institutional forces may either enhance or negate the development of multicultural competence. In other words, it does little good that service providers are culturally competent when the very organization that employs them is filled with monocultural policies and practices. In many cases, organizational customs do not value or allow the use of cultural knowledge or skills. Hospitals, insurance carriers, and both private and public agencies may even actively discourage, negate, or punish multicultural expressions. Thus, it is imperative to view multicultural competence for organizations as well. Developing new rules, regulations, policies, practices and structures within organizations, that enhance multiculturalism developing is important.

Overcoming Ethnocentric Monoculturalism: Professional Development

The traditional doctor-patient helping role may be severely culture-bound and not necessarily the most helpful one for persons of color. Multicultural theory stresses the importance of multiple helping roles developed by many culturally different groups and societies (Atkinson, Thompson, & Grant, 1993). Besides the basic one-on-one encounter aimed at curing the patient, alternative roles often involve larger social units, systems intervention, and prevention. That is, the conventional role of health care is only one of many others available to the helping professional.

Culturally competent helping is related to several factors (D.W. Sue, Carter et al., 1998). First, health care professionals must be able to free themselves from the confining Euro American definitions of service provision. Conventional helping roles are culture-bound and potentially unhelpful or oppressive to culturally different clients. Second, providers must begin to expand the range of their helping behaviors. Most service providers are products of medical or public health training programs, which are governed by standards of practice and codes of ethics that prescribe a very narrow band of behaviors or roles considered to be appropriate. Third, culturally relevant helping demands a broader range of helping roles played by the provider. The one-to-one doctor-patient session conducted in a sterile office, far removed from the real world, and aimed primarily at remediation may be ineffective when the source of problems reside in the environment (i.e., culturally sanctioned behaviors, community belief systems or the continuing impact of racism). Fourth, familiarity and skill in non-Western indigenous forms of healing contributes much to the multicultural-competent helping professional. Last, there is a need for health care providers to understand and be able to intervene on a larger systemic basis by creating multicultural agencies.

Developing Alternative Service Provider Roles

In Euro American society, being a professional health care provider is influenced by the values, knowledge base and beliefs of our society. Since the theories of health care originate from a particular cultural context, they also reflect those biases, in definitions of health and illness, human behavior, and the goals and processes of service delivery.

As a result, the standards for providers of services are unavoidably infused with primarily Eurocentric cultural values and assumptions. They may be applicable to one cultural group, but when applied to another, may constitute cultural oppression. Different cultural groups have different definitions or beliefs about what constitutes a helping relationship. Among Asian and many Asian American groups, for example, a helping relationship characterized by the following attributes: (1) subtlety and indirectness in communications, (2) vertical or hierarchical communication patterns, (3) respect for authority figures, and (4) the giving of advice and directions by a perceived expert. These characteristics may be at odds with those perceived by another culture as evidence of help.

In mental health practice, for example, the client is expected to be the more active of the participants; the giving of advice and directions is a traditional taboo; interpretation and confrontation is often used; the relationship between therapist and client is more egalitarian. For many Asian-American clients, the helpful therapist may be one who gives advice and suggestions, avoids confrontation and direct interpretation of motives and actions, indirectly discusses personal issues, does more initial talking than the client, and evidences a formal interactive approach. Traditional Asian American clients may attribute low credibility and expertise to a Euro American trained counselor or therapist. These therapeutic responses or approaches may be lacking in the behavioral repertoire of mental health professionals because they have not been trained to see helping in such a manner. Thus, even if they see the necessity of such an approach, they may feel uncomfortable in altering their characteristic style of helping.

Likewise, it is becoming clear that health care is also embedded in the wider sociopolitical forces of our society. Issues of race relations and the power differentials existing between different groups in our society are often played out in the helping relationship. Because the history of the United States is very much tied in to the oppressive treatment of racial/ethic minorities, many culturally different clients may enter the therapeutic relationship with great suspicion and wariness. They are likely to approach the helping professional with the following questions and thoughts: "What makes you any different from other White folds who have oppressed me?" "What makes you immune from inheriting the racial biases of your forebears?" "Why should I trust you?" "How open and honest are you about your biases?" "Before I open up to you, I need to know where you're coming from."

Racial/ethnic minorities and other oppressed groups are not likely to test the helping professional, to ascertain the answers to the above questions, and to make a decision regarding the trustworthiness of the helper. The testing may be quite overt and direct such as confronting the helper with the question "Are you a racist?" to more subtle statements such as "Most people could care less about minorities." Depending how the professional deals with these challenges will either enhance or diminish the trustworthiness of the service provider. A helping professional who fails to address directly the first question or chooses not to express a personal thought about the latter statement may seriously impair his or her credibility. In addition, a failure to adequately deal with these tests means the culturally different client will not self-disclose his or her most intimate thoughts and feelings.

Cultural flexibility in helping, expanding the repertoire of helping responses, and reconceptualizing the helping relationship in culturally relevant terms may truly enhance expertise, attractiveness and trustworthiness (APA, 1993). The use of nontraditional methods (music, ritual, dance, food, art, folk tales, etc.) to enhance a relationship may prove valuable, especially if it is culturally linked. Because health care providers are increasingly being asked to work with culturally different clients, and because they now realize that the conventional one-to-one, in-the-office, objective-form of treatment, aimed at remediation of existing problems may be at odds with the sociopolitical and cultural dimensions of their clients, they are finding their traditional therapeutic roles ineffective.

Three key forces are behind this trend. First, culturally different groups may not perceive or respond well to conventional treatment roles. Second, the locus of the problem may reside outside (external) rather than inside (internal) the client. For example, prejudice and discrimination like racism, sexism and homophobia may impede the healthy functioning of individuals and groups in our society. Third, is the impact of nonwestern or indigenous forms of healing.

Alternative roles to the conventional behavior care share certain characteristics:

(a) They are generally in the more active helping style of the provider;
(b) They often involve the provider working outside the office at the home, institution, or community of the client;
(c) The role of the provider is more externally focused and directed toward changing environmental conditions such as policies and practices of an organization, enhancing job opportunities, etc., as opposed to focusing on and changing the client;
(d) Clients are not perceived as having a problem (internal pathology), but as experiencing one (problematic situations);
(e) The alternative roles are more prevention-oriented as opposed to being primarily remediation in nature; and
(f) The provider shoulders an increased responsibility for determining the course and outcome of the helping process.

Some of these alternative roles are conceptually described below (Atkinson, Morten, & Sue, 1998; Atkinson, Thompson, & Grant, 1993). Note that they do not deny the importance of the conventional clinical roles, but rather see the following as complementary ones.

1. Advisor.   The main tasks of an advisor involve helping clients to solve or prevent potential health problems, educate them about available options, and sharing with them what they may found effective in dealing with the problematic situation. Immigrants, for example, may have minimal health care experience in U.S. society, and might benefit immensely from advice and suggestions.

2. Advocate. The role entails representing the individual's or group's best interests to other individuals groups, or institutions. They may, for example, represent a person who does not speak English well, and argue on their behalf for fair and equitable medical treatment. The role is not a neutral one and can entail political dimensions.

3. Consultant. This is a professional but collegial relationship in which both the helper and consultee work to impact or change a third party which may be related to policies of an organization or public health policy. Understanding of organizational dynamics and processes understanding is a necessity for this role.

4. Change Agent. The provider takes an action-oriented approach to changing aspects of the client's environment deemed to be unhealthy or to result in inferior care. In many respects this is similar to the consultant role, but the provider goes farther in assuming responsibility for making changes that may be oppressing clients or groups.

5. Facilitator of Indigenous Support Systems. Providers in this role realize that culturally different clients may respond better to indigenous support systems (the Church, extended family, community elders, indigenous healing methods, etc.) in resolving their problems. They refer out or place people in contact with the cultural resources available in the community.

6. Facilitator of Indigenous Healing Systems. Such a helper may take two courses of action: (a) refer clients to traditional healers such as a currandismo [Mexican folk healer] or Tai Chi Ch'uan instructor or (b) actually treating the client via indigenous healing methods. This latter action, however, assumes the provider is skilled and knowledgeable in those healing arts.

Learning from Indigenous Models of Healing

Ever since the beginning of human existence, all societies and cultural groups have developed not only their own explanations of illness and health, but also their culture specific ways of dealing with human problems and distress (Harner, 1990; Lee & Armstrong, 1995). Western forms of health, for example, rely on sensory information defined by the physical plane of reality (Western science), while most indigenous methods rely on the spiritual plane of existence in seeking a cure (Highlen, 1994, 1996). Western healing has failed to acknowledge or learn from these age-old forms of wisdom. Yet, in its attempt to become culturally responsive, the field of health care must begin to put aside the biases of Western science, to acknowledge the existence of intrinsic help-giving networks, and to incorporate the legacy of ancient wisdom, which may be contained in indigenous models of healing.

The Universal Shamanic Tradition, which encompasses the centuries-old recognition of healers within a community, continues to be influential in many minority communities (Lee, 1996; Lee, Oh, & Mountcastle, 1992). The anthropological term "Shaman" refers to people often called witch, witch doctor, wizard, medicine man or woman, sorcerer or magic man or woman. These individuals are believed to possess the power to enter an altered stated of consciousness and, in their healing rituals, journey to other planes of existence beyond the physical world. In a study of indigenous healing in 16 nonwestern countries, it was found that three approaches were often used (Lee, Oh, & Mountcastle, 1992).

First, there is heavy reliance on the use of communal, group and family networks to shelter the disturbed individual (Saudi Arabia), to problem solve in a group context

(Nigeria), and to reconnect them with family or significant others (Korea). Second, spiritual and religious beliefs and traditions of the community are used in the healing process. The reading of verses from the Koran and/or use of religious houses/churches are examples. Third, use of shamans (called piris and fakirs in Pakistan and Sudan) who are perceived to be the keepers of timeless wisdom is the norm.

Within these approaches are embedded some valuable lessons for behavioral health change.

1. Holistic Outlook on Life.   Most nonwestern indigenous forms of healing take a holistic outlook on well being in that they make minimal distinction between physical and mental functioning. The interrelatedness of life forms, the environment and the cosmos is a given. Illness, distress or problematic behavior is seen as an imbalance of internal or external forces. The seeking of harmony or balance is the healer's goal. Among American Indians, for example, harmony is symbolized by the circle, or hoop of life. Mind, body, spirit and nature are seen as a single unified entity with little separation between the realities of life, medicine and religion (Heinrich, Corbin, & Thomas, 1990). All forms of nature, not just the living, are to be revered because they reflect the creator or deity. Illness is seen as a break in the hoop of lie, an imbalance or separation between the elements. Likewise, the Afrocentric perspective with its roots in Egypt and Nubia teaches that human beings are part of a holistic fabric and should be oriented toward collective rather than individual survival (Asante, 1987). The indigenous Japanese assumptions and practices of Naikan and Morita therapy attempt to move clients toward being more in tune with others and society, to move away from individualism, and to move toward interdependence and connectedness (harmony with others).

2. The Importance of Spirituality in Being.   The United States has had a long tradition in believing that one's religious beliefs should not enter into scientific or rational decisions. Incorporating religion in health care treatment has generally been seen as unscientific and unprofessional. The schism occurred between religion and science centuries ago resulting in a split between science and religion (Highlen, 1994). This is often reflected in the phrase "separation of Church and State." The separation has become a serious barrier to Western medicine professionals incorporating indigenous forms of healing into their work, especially when religion is confused with spirituality. While all people may not have a formal religion, indigenous helpers believe that spirituality is an intimate aspect of the human condition. While western science acknowledges the behavioral, cognitive and affective realms, it only makes passing reference to the spiritual realm of existence. Yet, indigenous helpers believe that spirituality transcends time and space, transcends mind and body and transcends our behaviors, thoughts and feelings.

3. Journeys to Different Planes of Reality.   Intrinsic to the Universal Shamanic Tradition is the belief in the existence of different levels or planes of consciousness or experience (Hamer, 1990). Understanding and ameliorating the causes of illness or problems of life are often found in a different plane of reality rather than the physical world of existence. These non-ordinary reality states are the domain of the spirit world and it is believed that human destiny is often decided here. Shamans or indigenous helpers often enter these realities on behalf of their clients to seek answers to enlist the help of the spirit world, or to aid in realigning the spiritual energy field, which surrounds the body and extends throughout the universe. Ancient Chinese methods of healing and the Hindu chakra work, acknowledges another world of ethnic reality, which parallels the physical one (D.W. Sue & Sue, 1999; Highlen, 1996). Accessing this world allows the healer to use these special energy centers to balance and heal the body and mind. Occasionally, the

Shaman may aid the helpee or novice in accessing that plane of reality, so that he or she may find the solutions (Das, 1987; Karkar, 1982).

The vision quest in conjunction with the sweat lodge experience was used by American Indians as religious renewal or a rite of passage (Heinrich, Corbin, & Thomas, 1990). Behind these uses, however, is the human journey to another world of reality. The ceremony of the vision quest is intended to prepare the young man for the proper frame of mind: use of rituals and sacred symbols, prayers to the Great Spirit, isolation, fasting and personal reflection. Whether in a dream state of in full consciousness, another world of reality is said to reveal itself. Hindu mantras, chants, meditation and the taking of certain drugs (peyote) all have as their purpose to allow a journey into another world of existence.

In general, indigenous healing methods have much to offer to EuroAmerican forms of behavioral health care. The contributions are not only valuable because of the multiple belief systems that now exist in our society, but our health care agencies have neglected to deal with he spiritual dimension of human existence. Our heavy reliance on science and the reductionistic approach to treating clients have made us view human beings and human behavior as composed of separate non-interacting parts. There has been a failure to recognize our spiritual being and to take a holistic outlook on life. Indigenous models of healing remind us of these shortcomings and challenge us to look for answers in other realms of existence besides the physical world.

Conclusions

Culturally competent health care means massive and revolutionary changes in the health care industry. It means our ability to understand and accept the lived realities of the minority community. As such, it means change at the individual, professional, organizational and societal levels. Health care professionals must (1) take responsibility for attacking structural inequities which exist in our society (unequal distribution of wealth which results in minorities receiving medical help less frequently and at larger stages of illness, underserved communities, lack of health insurance, etc.), (2) monitor themselves with respect to racial stereotyping and biased assumptions about human behavior, (3) respect indigenous healing practices and build upon them to help minority constituents, and (4) develop their own cultural competence in relating to persons of color. As long as the racial divide in heath care exists, the quality of life for minority groups will continue to be poor, and their illness and mortality rates will remain higher than that of their white counterparts.

References

American Psychological Association. (1993). Guidelines for providers of psychological services to ethnic, linguistic, and culturally diverse populations. *American Psychologist*, 48, 45–48.

Asante, M. (1987). *The Afrocentric Idea*. Philadelphia: Temple University Press.

Atkinson, D.R., Morten, G., & Sue, D.W. (1998). *Counseling American Minorities*. New York: McGraw-Hill.

Atkinson, D.R., Thompson, C.E., & Grant, S.K. (1993). A three-dimensional model for counseling racial/ethnic minorities. *The Counseling Psycholcgist*.

Carter, R.T. (1995). *The Influence of Race and Racial Identity in Psychotherapy*. New York: John Wiley.

Clark, R., Anderson, N.B., Clark, V.R., & Williams, D.R. (1999). Racism as a stressor for African Americans: a biopsychosocial model. *American Psychologist*, 54, 805–816.

Das, A.K. (1987). Indigenous models of therapy in traditional Asian societies. *Journal of Multicultural Counseling and Development*, 15, 25–37.

Hall, C.T. (1999). Study finds racial divide in lung cancer treatments. *San Francisco Chronicle*, October 14, 1999, pp. Al, A6.

Harner, M. (1990). *The Way of the Shaman*. San Francisco: Harper and Row.

Heinrich, R.K., Corbin, J.L., & Thomas, K.R. (1990). Counseling Native Americans. *Journal of Counseling and Development*, 69, 128–133.

Herring, R.D. (1997). *Counseling Diverse Ethnic Youth*. Fort Worth, TX: Harcourt Brace.

Highlen, P.S. (1994). Racial/ethnic diversity in doctoral programs of psychology: challenges for the twenty-first century. *Applied and Preventive Psychology*, 3, 91–108.

Highlen, P.S. (1996). MCT theory and implications for organizations/systems. In D.W. Sue, A.E. Ivey, & P.B. Pedersen (Eds.), *A Theory of Multicultural Counseling and Therapy* (pp. 65–85). Pacific Grove, CA: Brooks Cole.

Hoshmand, L.S.T. (1989). Alternate research paradigms: a review and teaching proposal. *The Counseling Psychologist*, 17, 3–79.

Jones, J.M. (1997). *Prejudice and Racism*. 2nd Edition. New York: McGraw-Hill.

Kakar, S. (1982). *Shamans, Mystics and Doctors: A Psychological Inquiry into India and Its Healing Traditions*. New York: Knopf.

Lee, C.C. (1996). MCT theory and implications for indigenous healing. In D. Sue, A.E. Ivey, and P.B. Pedersen (Eds.), *A Theory of Multicultural Counseling and Therapy*. Pacific Grove, CA: Brooks Cole.

Lee, C.C. & Armstrong, K.L. (1995). Indigenous models of mental health intervention: lessons from traditional healers. In J.G. Ponterotto, J.M. Casas, L.A. Suzuki, & C.M. Alexander, (Eds.), *Handbook of multicultural counseling*, pp. 441–456. Thousand Oaks, CA: Sage.

Lee, C.C., Oh, M.Y., & Mountcastle, A.R. (1992). Indigenous models of helping in nonwestern countries: Implications for multicultural counseling. *Journal of Multicultural Counseling and Development*, 20, 1–10.

Parham, T.A., White, J.L., & Ajamu, A. (1999). *The Psychology of Blacks*. Upper Saddle River, NJ: Prentice Hall.

President's Initiative on Race. (1998). *One America in the 21st Century*.

Sue, D.W., Arredondo, P., & McDavis, R.J. (1992). Multicultural competencies/standards: a pressing need. *Journal of Counseling and Development*, 70(4), 477–486.

Sue, D.W., Carter, R.T., Casas, J.M., Fouad, N.A., Ivey, A.E., Jensen, M., Lafromboise, T., Manese, J.E., Ponterotto, J.G., & Vazquez-Nutall, E. (1998). *Multicultural Counseling Competencies: Individual and Organizational Development*. Thousand Oaks, CA: Sage.

Sue, D.W., & Sue, D. (1999). *Counseling the Culturally Different: Theory and Practice*. New York: Wiley.

U.S. Census Bureau. (1992). *Statistical Abstract of the United States*. The National Data Book (112th Ed.) Washington, DC: Bureau of The Census.

U.S. Department of Health and Human Services. (1985). *Report of the Secretary's Task Force on Black and Minority Health*. Washington, D.C.: U.S. Government Printing Office.

Williams, D.R., & Collins, C. (1995). US socioeconomic and racial differences in health: patterns and explanations. *Annual Review of Sociology*, 21, 349–386.

Williams, D.R., Lavizzo-Mourey, R., & Warren, R.C. (1994). The concept of race and health status in America. *Public Health Reports*, 109, 26–41.

Chapter **4**

Prevention Science
Theory, Research, and Implications for Practice

WARREN A. RHODES, ROLANDE MURRAY, AND MARLENE GREER-CHASE

According to a recent report (National Academy Press, 1994), nearly one third of American adults will suffer from a diagnosable mental disorder during their lifetime and, even more significant, nearly 20% will have a disorder at any given time (p. xi). Unfortunately, there is an insufficient pool of well-trained prevention researchers who study the causes and prevention of mental disorders.

The need to train more prevention researchers is included in the recent recommendations of three national scientific mental health advisory committee reports: the *National Institute of Mental Health Report; the Prevention of Mental Disorders: A National Research Agenda* and the *Institute of Medicine Report, Reducing Risks for Mental Disorders: Frontiers for Preventive Intervention Research;* and *Priorities for Prevention Research at NIMH.* These reports represent a national agenda for research efforts aimed at the prevention of mental disorders, and are the culmination of several years of scientific investigation and review. According to one report, a major barrier to development of the prevention field is the slow pace of developing scientists for prevention research (National Advisory Mental Health Council Report, May 15, 1995).

It is generally agreed that minorities are over-represented in the incidence of mental disorders. Unfortunately, they are under-represented in the ranks of research professionals in the field of prevention of these disorders. The need for well-trained minority prevention researchers has been declared:

> In addition, a major increase in the training of ethnic minority prevention researchers is needed…Many more minority investigators than are currently supported should receive training in prevention research, and a similar number of minority undergraduate students should be involved in outreach activities to recruit them for training in prevention research. (Ibid.)

Without question, the pace of training minority prevention scientists is woefully slow. There must be a comprehensive and sustained effort directed toward increasing the number of minority prevention researchers. With this in mind, the Morgan State University

Prevention Science Training program is designed to increase the number of minority investigators in the pipeline, training for a specialty in prevention science.

To increase the numbers of African-Americans who obtain advanced degrees in the important area of prevention science, Baltimore City Public Schools, Morgan State University, and the Prevention Research Center at John Hopkins School of Hygiene and Public Health together developed an interdisciplinary prevention science research-training program in public mental health. The program goals are centered on a multidisciplinary approach to training Morgan State University students majoring in biology, education, psychology, and social work to conduct effective, meaningful prevention research and programming consistent with the recommendations of national advisory reports.

Specifically, the Institute of Medicine's report (National Academy Press, 1994) suggests that effective and meaningful preventive intervention research training requires direct experience in established institutions or centers carrying out prevention studies (p. 460). The Morgan State University Prevention Science Training Program functions as an integral part of the ongoing prevention research of the Hopkins Prevention Research Center, beginning with the periodic follow-up of over 2300 youths from East Baltimore City public elementary schools who have been assessed annually since 1984 and 1985, when they were randomly assigned to preventive intervention trials in first and second grade. This epidemiologically defined sample represents the first generation of Baltimore preventive intervention trials. The Institute of Medicine's report stated, "The trainee's experience should include participation in all phases of an actual preventive intervention research program that is being conducted by faculty of the training institution ... The trainee's mentors need to have had actual experience in one or more phases of design and analysis, and at least some of them should be actively engaged in such tasks during a trainee's participation. A clear implication is that the training-institution itself must be actively engaged in a continuing program of preventive intervention research, perhaps with shifting emphases and different types of intervention, but steadily engaged." (p. 460)

The collaboration with Johns Hopkins Prevention Research Center, a major prevention research training institution, affords Morgan State University faculty and students the benefits of a well-established prevention research training mechanism, including a wealth of knowledge, expertise and resources.

Theoretical Orientation for Prevention Science

While much has been learned about the causes, diagnosis and treatment of mental disorders, much less is known about the prevention of these disorders. The prevention of mental disorders is a public health goal that originated more than a century ago. However, in the past several decades there has been a renewed interest in the prevention of these disorders (National Academy Press, 1994). If the prevention of mental health problems is to become a reality and not just an admirable goal for those interested in improving mental health outcomes for our citizens, we must develop an understanding of both risk and protective factors. We must understand the factors that predispose children to healthy, as well as unhealthy, mental outcomes. Not only must we understand what factors facilitate or hinder various mental health outcomes, but also we must know for whom these factors have an effect and why. Prevention science is an emerging field in public mental health that provides the framework to systematically understand both protective and risk factors associated with various mental health conditions. Prevention science is interdisciplinary, incorporating sociological, developmental, epidemiological, and psychological perspectives of mental health problems. Prevention scientists may be trained as community psychologists, epidemiologists, sociologists, psychiatrists or even economists.

Prevention Science Framework

Prevention science framework involves combining three major research orientations: *life-course development, community epidemiology, and experimental preventive intervention trials.*

Life-Course Developmental Orientation

Life-course development orientation suggests that most humans move through very distinct stages of life, and that current and future behaviors, including maladaptive behaviors and related disorders, are determined by significant factors that occur at various periods during development. Life-course developmental orientation has afforded the opportunity for researchers to map the developmental paths that lead to various health outcomes.

Community Epidemiology

Prevention science embraces the concept that maladaptive outcomes vary within a community and that one can study and understand what factors contribute to the variation. Prevention science researchers study a specifically defined population in environments such as the family, neighborhood, and/or community. When general characteristics, such as poverty and ethnicity, are held constant, major factors that explain the variation in health outcomes are then examined. When coupled with the life-course development framework, community epidemiology allows for the study of individuals who develop poor health outcomes, and compares them to those in the same community who do not. A prevention science perspective determines what factors seem important in differentiating those who exhibit the maladaptive behavior from those who do not.

Preventive Intervention Trials

Using an epidemiologically defined population, preventive intervention trials determine the effectiveness of an intervention by targeting factors believed to have impact on various health outcomes. In addition to providing evidence of the impact of specific interventions on poor health outcomes, for example, preventive intervention trials can help to clarify whether we can change the course of maladaptive outcomes. Using the prevention science framework, Sheppard Kellam and his colleagues at the Johns Hopkins Prevention Research Center continue to demonstrate and discuss how prevention science can affect the course and malleability of maladaptive outcomes, including drug abuse and related disorders (See for example, Kellam, 1983; Kellam & Rebok, 1992; Kellam & Van Horn, 1997; Kellam, Ling, Merisca, Brown, Rubin, Ensminger & Lalongo, 1998).

Morgan State University Prevention Science Training Program

The training of Morgan State University students in prevention science occurs within the existing Johns Hopkins Prevention Research Program, using the first generation prevention research protocol and focusing on the prevention and malleability of maladaptive behaviors. This training consists of three major components: *summer research training experience, year-long research training assistantship, and biweekly honors seminars.*

Summer Research Training Experience

The Johns Hopkins Prevention Research Center employed students in the capacity of "field assessors". As part of this research training program, each student received work/training experience totaling 240 hours over the course of the summer. The research training began with an intensive protocol to orient students to prevention science methods, in general, and to the Prevention Research Center's underlying theoretical framework, in particular. Training was conducted in a seminar format with formal presentations by program staff, including Drs. Sheppard Kellam, Warren Rhodes, and Rolande Murray, and incorporated informal discussions with students, which facilitated their acquisition of prevention science knowledge. Additionally, students were required to read prevention science research literature (e.g., Kellam & Rebok, 1992; Kellam & Van Horn, 1997) and to make well-articulated presentations to fellow students and program scientists. The initial training included the following areas of concentration:

- Overview and History of the Prevention Science Partnership
- Developmental Epidemiology-Based Prevention Science
- Prevention Science Periodic Follow-Up: Data and Collection Methods
- Interview, Clinical Observation, Neuropsychologic and Physiologic Measures
- Developmental Epidemiology and Multi-Stage Sampling Techniques
- Participant Tracking
- Confidentiality and Informed Consent
- Crisis Response
- Ongoing Supervision and Mentoring.

During the remainder of the summer, students participated in hands-on research activities. For example, students worked on revising and editing the assessment instruments used in the follow-up fieldwork; some students worked on tracking research participants, while others worked on computerizing the assessment instruments. While most of the research activities were new experiences for the students, some activities allowed them to strengthen their research skills using real data sets. For example, some students had the opportunity to enhance their statistical skills using SPSS and SAS; all students gained some computer experience, including the use of computer graphics such as PowerPoint and CorelDraw for presentations.

All students were provided ongoing progress evaluations. At the conclusion of the eight-week summer training experience, they were either recommended or not recommended to continue with the program for the upcoming academic year.

Year-Long Research Training Assistantship

Many tasks were associated with the periodic follow-up using the longitudinal, epidemiologically defined population of 2,300. Measures had to be defined, standardized collection procedures established, and reliability and validity checks made. A primary reason this research training experience was found to be so beneficial to students was that, as the research protocol unfolded, students were able to participate in a variety of activities supporting the research process. At the beginning of the research training experience, students were instrumental in getting the follow-up ready for the field. They received hands-on research experience including:

- revising and editing the assessment instrument for the field,
- tracking participants with whom the Prevention Program had lost contact,
- computerizing the assessment instruments,
- designing and researching relevant stories for the program newsletter,
- writing drafts of initial contact letters sent to the study population, and
- working with other researchers in the Program to help format data for analysis using statistical packages such as SPSS and SAS.

Every effort was made to ensure that all students had an opportunity to participate in each activity. Since computerized data collection was a significant component of the research protocol, a considerable amount of research training time was focused on field training in that area.

Field Training

In preparation for the field interview of the 2,300 young adults, students received intense interviewer training. The interview training involved every student progressing through the entire assessment instrument, which at the time was four hours long. Students were led in the role-playing of both interviewer and interviewee. Students were also given the opportunity to observe dyad interactions and provide critical feedback.

Biweekly Honors Seminar Training Component

As part of the training program, students were required to attend a biweekly honors seminar and at least one Prevention Science Forum lecture series sponsored by the Prevention Research Center (PRC). The objective of the seminars was to bring into perspective the students' hands-on research experience at PRC, with an understanding of how the research experience was related to public health and, specifically, to prevention science. The students' research training experiences were structured around such topics as community base-building, ethics and research, roles and responsibilities, tracking in the field, and conducting research in the community.

To further build on the collaborative aspects and partnership with other prevention research sites, all students became affiliate members of Early Career Preventionist Network (ECPN). Moreover, students were encouraged to attend local and national symposia and conferences related to public health and prevention science. Such participation included:

- A one-day symposium on *Urban Health Issues for the 21st Century*, sponsored by the Morgan State University Public Health Planning Program and the Institute for Urban Research.

- A trip to Tempe, Arizona to participate in the Second Biannual Conference on Minority Issues in Prevention Science, sponsored by Arizona State University's Preventive Intervention Research Center, where students participated in a panel discussion.
- The Sixth Annual Meeting of the Society for Prevention Research, held in Park City, Utah, a multidisciplinary conference that presented students with new research advancements from a variety of prevention research disciplines, including alcohol abuse, tobacco use, illicit drug use, and mental health problems.
- A meeting and formal presentation to the Morgan State University Prevention Science Steering Committee (PSSC), discussing their experience working in the prevention science research field and their expectations for the future as scientists.

As the academic mentor and Associate Science Director of the Prevention Program, Dr. Murray worked very closely with each student in researching graduate training programs. Dr. Murray provided resources and support to the students for preparing their graduate school personal statements, for contacting faculty members and other research scientists at prospective graduate schools, and for acquiring any other information that would help them gain access to graduate programs related to public health.

What Are the Paths Taken by Prevention Research Science Trainees?

We are very encouraged to note that the students' experience in the Prevention Program had significant impact on their future professional direction. Six seniors participated in the training program in the first year; all six are on track to begin careers related to public health and, in particular, to prevention science. For example, one student entered a Ph.D. program at the Prevention Research Center at Arizona State University, while another went on to pursue an MSW, with an emphasis on prevention, at Howard University. Three students remained with the Prevention Program at Johns Hopkins to gain further prevention science experience. Specifically, one student trained in phlebotomy and neuropsychological assessments and worked as an XRF Lead Technician for a lead grant supplemental study, while another student assumed the role of Coordinator of Field Operations on the grant entitled *Periodic Follow-up of Two Universal Preventive Trials*, (R01MH57005) with Dr. Nicholas Ialongo as Principal Investigator.

The Changing Face of the Undergraduate Minority Training Program in Prevention Science

As students progressed in the prevention science training program they were provided advanced training opportunities. That is, all students moved into another phase of the training Program: *Prevention Science Workgroup* and Mini-Workgroups, where they received one-to-one mentoring from prevention research faculty. The larger Prevention Science Workgroup is a structured network of local (e.g., Morgan State, Johns Hopkins and Towson University) and remote (e.g., University of South Florida and Michigan State University) research collaborators. The Prevention Science Workgroup meets weekly in a forum where the various mini-research group participants present' and discuss ongoing research projects, manuscripts and/or grants in preparation. Another feature of this larger workgroup is that it provides collaborators with a forum to present new research ideas that may not yet have taken shape. All students attended the larger prevention science workgroup.

As participants in the mini-workgroups, students learned specific statistical analysis tools, such as growth curve modeling, imputations, power analysis, and person analysis. They were active participants in planning next-stage intervention trials, reviewing drafts of manuscripts, doing literature reviews, and participating in rewrites and edits of manuscripts and/or grants. Drs. Marlene Greer-Chase, Warren A. Rhodes, and Sheppard Kellam led a mini-workgroup that focused on teacher training as a potential preventive intervention to reduce aggressive, disruptive classroom behaviors. A brief description of this workgroup follows.

Mini-Workgroup: Level of Discipline in Public Schools and the Need for Classroom Management Skills

There is a large literature in developmental psychopathology, which informs us on the course of maladaptive behaviors, and supports a research focus on the nature and development of classroom disciplinary problems. We suggest that some important insight into the long-standing disciplinary problems observed in our public schools may lie in an understanding of the development, course and malleability of aggressive behaviors that have been uncovered through extensive research in the broad area of developmental psychopathology. For example, we have clear evidence that maladaptive aggressive responses (breaking rules, truancy, and fighting) to classroom social demands, occurring as early as first grade, predict a host of maladaptive behaviors, including antisocial behavior, criminality, and heavy intravenous drug use later in life. Along these lines, research suggests the lack of effective disciplinary procedures in the elementary school classroom—procedures that curtail aggressive behaviors—may have important developmental consequences, including future maladaptive behaviors.

Growing concern that a number of the nation's teachers are underqualified to teach our children has focused attention on the quality of their pre-service learning, and especially on the institutions that prepare prospective teachers.

Blum (1994) found that despite the plethora of classroom management materials available to teachers, many remain inadequate in their classroom management skills. In the findings of this study, Blum reported that pre-service teachers do not receive comprehensive training in classroom/school management from their teacher education programs.

At this point our study group questioned, why do teachers not receive adequate training in classroom management skills? How can we better assure that pre-service teachers are given the necessary tools for more effective classroom management? One reason teachers may not receive adequate classroom management skills is that National Council of Accreditation of Teacher Education (NCATE) standards do not mandate specific evaluation to determine whether teacher education programs are providing both theoretical and practical classroom management training for the pre-service teacher, even though the literature is replete with research-based demands for specific and direct instruction in classroom management at the pre-service level.

Knowing the results from research conducted by Kellam and colleagues, various education researchers (e.g. Blum, 1994; Jones, 1996), and the National Commission on Teaching and America's Future (NCTAF), this workgroup, in conjunction with the Morgan State University Department of Education, proposed to investigate how we can better assure that teachers are given the management tools proven to be most effective in the classroom.

Implications for Practice

As a comprehensive university, Morgan State University recognizes the strong, symbiotic relationship between quality teaching, research, and public service. The University emphasizes quality teaching at all levels and ensures that research and service capabilities and resources enhance the instructional component of its mission. Morgan ranks among the top campuses nationally in preparation of African-American students for advanced study, and is designated by legislative statue as Maryland's "Public Urban University." As such, it gives priority to addressing the needs of the populations of urban areas, and is committed to increasing educational attainment of the African-American population in fields and at degree levels in which it is underrepresented.

In December 1998, the Maryland Higher Education Commission approved the Master of Public Health/Doctor of Public Health degree, making Morgan the first historically Black university to offer a doctorate in public health. While this public health degree program is practice-oriented and specifically designed to train students in the application of public health knowledge and skills, it will draw upon the public mental health research training that the current prevention program is designed to cultivate. The current prevention science training program strengthen Morgan's capabilities to train minorities in the discovery of prevention strategies for mental disorders, and inform mental health practitioners in the knowledge base and skills for successful intervention in the public health arena.

References

Blum, H. (1994). The pre-service teacher's educational training in classroom discipline: a national survey of teacher education programs. (Doctoral dissertation, Temple University Graduate Board). *Dissertation abstracts international. (UMI Dissertation Service. No. 9434650).*

Ensminger, M., Kellam, S., & Rubin, B. (1983). School and family origins of delinquency: comparison by sex. In K. Van Duse, S. Mednick, (Eds.), *Prospective Studies of Crime and Delinquency.* Boston: Kluwer-Nijhof, pp. 73–97.

Institute of Medicine. (1994). In P.J. Mrazek & R.J. Haggerty (Eds), *Reducing Risks for Metal Disorders: Frontiers for Preventive Intervention Research.* Washington, DC: National Academy Press.

Jones, V. (1996). Classroom management. In J.P. Sikula, T.J. Buttery, & E. Guyton (Eds.), *Handbook of Research on Teacher Education.* New York: Simon and Schuster Macmillan.

Kellam, S. (1990). Developmental epidemiologic framework for family research on depression and aggression. In G.R. Patterson (Ed.), *Depression and Aggression in Family Interaction.* Englewood Cliffs, NJ: Erlbaum pp. 11–48.

Kellam, S., Brown, C., Rubin, B., & Ensminger, M. (1983). Paths leading to teenage psychiatric symptoms and substance use: developmental epidemiological studies in Woodlawn. In S. Guze, F. Earls & J. Barrett (Eds.), *Childhood Psychopathology and Development.* New York: Raven Press, pp. 17–55.

Kellam, S., Ling, X., Merisca, R., Brown, C., & Lalongo, N. (1998). The effect of level of aggression in the first-grade classroom on the course and malleability of aggressive behavior into middle school. *Development and Psychopathology,* 10, 165–185.

Kellam, S. & Rebok, G. (1992). Building developmental and etiological theory through epidemiologically based preventive intervention trials. In J. McCord, & R.E. Tremblay (Eds.), *Preventing Anti-Social Behavior: Interventions from Birth through Adolescence.* New York: Guilford Press, pp. 162–195.

Kellam, S. & Van Horn, Y. (1997). Life course development, community epidemiology, and preventive trials: A scientific structure for prevention research. *American Journal of Community Psychology,* 25(2), 177–188.

Kellam, S., Werthamer-Larsson, L., Dolan, F., Brown, C., Mayer, L., Rebok, G., Anthony, A., Laudoff, J., & Edelsohn, G. (1991). Developmental epidemiologically based preventive trials: baseline modeling of early target behaviors and depressive symptoms. *American Journal of Community Psychology*, 19(4), pp. 563–584.

National Commission on Teaching and America's Future. (1997). *Doing What Matters Most: Investing In Quality Teaching*. New York: NCTAF.

National Council of Accreditation of Teacher Education. (1997). *Standards and Policies for the Accreditation of Professional Education Units*. Washington, DC: NCATE.

National Council of Accreditation of Teacher Education. (1996). *Teacher Preparation: A Guide to Colleges and Universities*. Washington, DC: NCATE.

National Institutes of Health, National Institute of Mental Health. (1998). Priorities for Prevention Research at NIMH: *A Report by the National Advisory Mental Health Council Workgroup on Mental Disorders Prevention Research*. Rockville, MD. Author.

National Institute of Mental Health. (1995). *A Plan for Prevention Research for the National Institute of Mental Health: A Report to the National Advisory Mental Health Council*.

Chapter **5**

Violence Prevention in African American Youth

WILLIAM B. LAWSON, JIMMY CUNNINGHAM, AND VALERIE LAWSON

Introduction

Youth violence is a significant problem in many American communities, particularly inner city communities, which have a disproportionately high African American population. Homicide is the leading cause of death among young African American men age 15 to 34 with rates six to seven times that of whites (Griffith & Bell 1989). Furthermore the amount of near lethal violence *is* many times that of the homicide rate. Violence is not equally distributed across all neighborhoods, but occurs disproportionately in inner city neighborhoods, among the young, and in public places (Bell & Jenkins, 1993). Violence is not a uniquely racial problem since the excess mortality is accounted for by social factors such as poverty and unemployment (Rosenberg et al., 1992; Runyan & Gerken, 1989). Nevertheless, violence and its consequences remain a major public health problem for the African American community (Griffith & Bell, 1989; Rosenberg et al., 1992).

Since violence is so prevalent in inner city neighborhoods, it is also often witnessed as well as experienced, partially because it is often public (Griffith & Bell, 1993; Richters & Martinez, 1993). One informal survey of ten mothers in a Chicago housing project found that all of the children had a firsthand encounter with a shooting by age 5 (Dubrow & Gabarino, 1989). Another study in inner city Chicago found that 26% of children in grades second through eight had witnessed someone being shot and 30% had witnessed a stabbing (Bell & Jenkins, 1993). Another survey of high school students found that 75% had witnessed a robbery, stabbing shooting, and/or killing, 35% had witnessed a stabbing, 39% a shooting, and 24% of someone being killed (Shakoor & Chalmers, 1991). A survey of grades 6 through 10 in New Haven showed that 40% witnessed at least one violent crime in the past year (Maras and Cohen, 1993). Pynoos and Eth (1985) estimated that children witness approximately 10 to 20% of the homicides committed in Los Angeles. Richters and Martinez (1993) reported that 72% of children 6–10 living in a low-income neighborhood in Washington, DC had witnessed violence. Osofsky et al. (1993) reported that

91% of African American children aged 9–12 in a low-income neighborhood in New Orleans had witnessed violence.

Exposure to violence may have substantial consequences. Parallels have been drawn between children growing up in inner cities in the United States and those "living in war zones," "living in battle zones," and "surviving in a battle free zone" (Bell & Jenkins, 1991; Lorion & Saltzman, 1993). Gabarino et al. (1991) noted similarities between the lives of children encountering urban violence and children living in combat areas. Effects of violence exposure tend to be cumulative and enduring, and include regressive behavior, feelings of helplessness, emotional numbness, and problems with attention and concentration leading to difficulties in academic performance (Bell & Jenkins, 1993; Pynoos & Nader, 1998). Moreover, distress symptoms are significantly correlated with violence exposure (Richter & Martinez, 1993).

Some of these violence-exposed children may meet criteria for posttraumatic stress disorder (PTSD), a phenomenon usually associated with combat veterans (Osofsky, 1995). Military experience had shown that combat veterans exposed to extraordinary stresses developed persistent symptoms long after the stressful situation had ceased. The phenomenology of PTSD included hallucinatory-like flashbacks, blunted emotional reactivity, hypervigilance, relationship difficulty, housing instability, employment problems, and substance abuse.

Recent research has demonstrated that PTSD occurs outside of the military situation. Victims of rape and child abuse, including sexual abuse and violence may also develop PTSD. McLeer reported high rates of PTSD in child sexual abuse victims. A retrospective study on inpatients at the Medical College of Pennsylvania (Deblinger et al., 1989) showed that 20.9% of sexually abused children and 6.9% of physically abused children met diagnostic criteria for PTSD. Interestingly, 10.3% of the nonabused group met criteria for PTSD. The PTSD in abused children has been associated with persisting symptoms. Symptoms ranged from depression and anxiety to behavioral disorders (Kiser, 1991). Criteria for the diagnosis of PTSD in adults are (1) exposure to an event that could be traumatic, (2) intrusive reexperiencing of the trauma, (3) numbing of responsiveness to or reducing involvement with the external world, and (4) two or more other symptoms (hyper-alertness/startle; sleep disturbance, survivor guilt, impaired memory/concentration, and intensification of symptoms when exposed to cues related to trauma.

Osofsky (1995) reviewed much of the relevant literature and concluded that traumatized elementary school children show behaviors similar to those seen in adult combat veterans, i.e., nightmares, preoccupation with the traumatic event, complex reenactment of the event, and appreciation of the irreversibility to the event. Finally, as noted above, youth witnessing urban violence or experiencing violence may either develop PTSD or show symptoms suggestive of PTSD, although most of the remote literature focused on combat veterans, and recent literature on abused children or extreme violence (Osofsky, 1995).

The recent literature provides clear evidence that experiencing urban violence may lead to outcomes as well as symptoms similar to those seen in combat veterans, abused children, and children experiencing extreme violence. They showed increased anxiety, depression, aggressiveness, and withdrawal (Freeman et al., 1993; Pynoos, 1993). Fighting and aggressive behavior may be one of the most common behavioral problems from exposure to urban violence (Durant et al., 1994; Pynoos, 1993; Shakoor & Chalmers, 1989). Boys in particular are more prone to seek weapons or want to use a weapon to resolve conflicts (Bell & Jenkins, 1993). Poor academic performance, including low grades, and school dropout are associated (Shakoor & Chalmers, 1989). Emotional numbing appears to be common as children and adults acted matter-of-factly or treated it as nothing special seeing a dead body or a shooting (Osofsky, 1995; Lorion & Saltzman, 1993). Youth in such neighborhoods also report significantly higher levels of exposure to drug-related activity, greater access and availability of drugs, and higher levels of current, lifetime, and intended drug and alcohol use (Lorion & Saltzman 1993). In fact, such children reported levels of drug and alcohol use up to ten times that of children living in neighborhoods with low levels of violent incidents.

Limited studies suggest possible positive interventions. Unfortunately, parenting may be compromised because parents also report helplessness and hopelessness (Richters & Martinez, 1993). The anxiety of caregivers in. these circumstances probably exacerbates the PTSD symptoms of the children (Osofsky et al., 1994). Interestingly, however, these children felt very safe at home and school, suggesting the importance of interventions involving parents or schools (Bell & Jenkins, 1993; Osofsky et al., 1994). Moreover, resilience factors, i.e., those associated with fewer negative symptoms, include having a supportive person in the environment, having a protected place, and having individual resources (Osofsky et al., 1994). Other resilience factors include having higher scores on a purpose of life scale, regular attending religious service, stress reduction, and positive parental support (Durant et al., 1994).

As noted above, much of the research in PTSD has involved combat veterans and abused children. Although exposure to violence has been associated with PTSD, there has been far less research in this area. More needs to be done to determine the prevalence of this problem in inner city areas outside of the major cities, to determine its relationship to poor school performance, anxiety, and depression, and most importantly to behaviors that create the "vicious cycle of violence," i.e., aggressiveness, violent behavior, drug use, and use of guns. More needs to be done to determine the similarity of the PTSD that develops in the youth to the PTSD seen in child abuse and combat veterans. Finally, there is little research on resilience factors and on the effectiveness of intervention programs in addressing these concerns.

Philander Smith College was granted a violence prevention project funded by the Office of Minority Health. The project involved enrichment and violence prevention programs that reduce the risk of violence through 19 Family Life Centers, based at Historically Black Colleges and Universities around the country. The director of the project is the last author of this chapter. The lead authors were invited to evaluate the effectiveness of the project. In the remainder of the chapter, the results of that evaluation will be discussed. Youth in this project were recruited from the central Little Rock, Arkansas area.

According to 1990 United States census data, Arkansas has a high rate of single parent families, is last in the nation in a number of health indicators, has high rates of AIDS and sexually transmitted diseases, low income, limited education resources, and a history of racial polarization; gun ownership is extensive and encouraged. According to FBI statistics, Little Rock has been consistently in the top ten in homicides in the nation for cities its size, had been number one during 1993, and in 1994 was the third most violent city in the nation. In 1993, the city, which has a population of less than 200,000, had 76 homicides, of which 50 were African American males, 27 under the age of 29 and most occurring in central city. A recent Home Box Office program that was aired nationally documented the high rate of homicide, gang violence, and related drug abuse in this midsize city. Gang activity is prevalent with over fifty known gangs. Los Angeles- and Chicago-based gangs have active chapters, including the Crips, Bloods, and Disciples. Youth in the program was drawn from a predominately central city community with high homicide rates, drive-by shootings, and high rates of arrests for drug abuse, especially crack cocaine. The community is flanked on one side by historical Central High School and the other by the downtown area.

The Family Life Center is a three-year comprehensive community-based project entitled "Brother to Brother" designed to (1) increase the resiliency and protective factors that place youth at-risk for alcohol and other drug-related violence and (2) to decrease the prevalence of drug use and accompanying violent acts among the target population. There are two programs involved: Project Spirit for ages 6–12, and Project Simba for ages 15–18. The program is housed at the Liberty Hill Missionary Baptist Church in the central Little Rock community described above.

The Programs

Education and Enrichment
- After-school instruction and tutoring, computer laboratory, reading incentives, career counseling

Discipline and Structure
- Reinforcement based, Tae-Kwon Do martial arts instruction/program
- Afrocentric base
- History instruction, tradition focused, rites of passage overlay

Parent Involvement
- Family nights, family outreach, parent education

Creative Recreation
- Tae Kwon Do, field trips
- Creativity and self-initiative encouraged

Creative Learning
- Rap sessions, Afrocentric tradition approaches

Community Outreach
- School and home visits by staff, a board of directors made up of community members, college student and parent volunteers
- Referral Services available to a mental health center.

The Participants

Fifty African American males were enrolled, 25 in Project Spirit and 25 in Project Simba. The criteria for enrollment were poor academic achievement, school behavioral problems, juvenile or criminal justice involvement, drug or alcohol use, and gang activity. The primary reason for enrollment included academics, 66.7%; behavior, 20.8%; gang involvement, 8.3%; and drug use 4.2%.

Evaluation Instruments

To evaluate violence and drug exposure, students were administered "Things I Have Seen and Heard" in which respondents indicated whether or not they were exposed to various

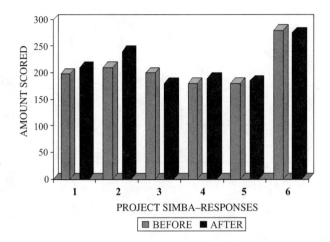

Figure 8.   African Self-Conscious Scale.

events, and "Levonn," in which respondents respond as to whether they can identify with a cartoon child expressing various responses to violent incidents (Richter and Martinez, 1993). Self-concept and identity was assessed with the African Self-Concept Scale (Figure 8), a scale developed and copyrighted by Joe Baldwin, Ph.D., at Florida A&M University. Grade point average was the primary performance outcome measure. This is a widely used scale to determine self-concept in African American youth as an aspect of their ethnic identity. It can be used to assess if the Afrocentric program specifically improves ethnic identity or self-concept in general.

Evaluation Procedure

Youth were evaluated within one month of entering the program and again six months later. Evaluations were done at the program site. A psychiatrist or psychologist was present to assist in the test administration and also to reassure youth distressed by the test items.

Results

The first group of figures is the responses for the Project Spirit participants. These are baseline results in which responders and nonresponders are counted. Figure 9 shows that a majority has heard gunshots in this metropolitan area.

Figure 10 shows that a significant number, approximately 20% of these young participants, have witnessed significant violence or its consequences.

The nonresponses parallel the responses, indicating that the nonresponders were not simply those that did not witness violence. Over half of participants reported at least one symptom. When asked why they did not respond, several of the participants stated that they had seen the HBO special and did not want to spoil the reputation of the community. Several participants were heard complaining, however, that these kinds of questions made them think of things they do not want to think about.

Rates of personal violence or specific violent threats are relatively low, but threats are high.

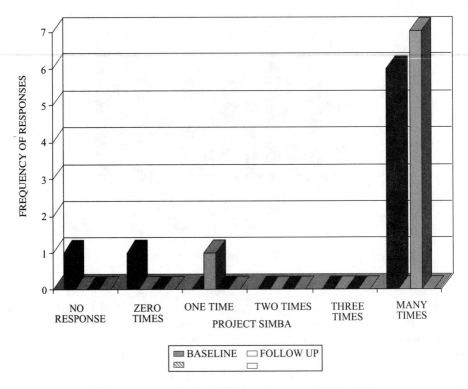

Figure 9.   Question 1: I have heard guns being shot—Project Spirit.

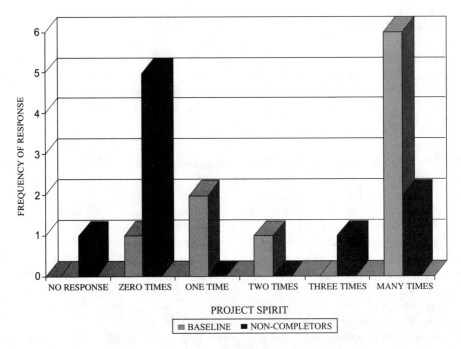

Figure 10.   Question 5: I have seen somebody being beat up.

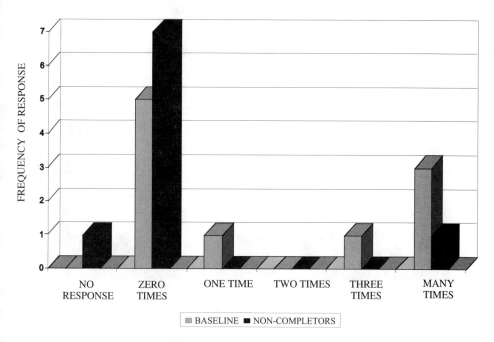

Figure 11.   I feel safe when I am at school.

Reports of domestic violence or illegal activity at home are relatively low, but threats appear common. Not surprisingly, they report feeling safer at school than the home (Figure 11). Nevertheless, a substantial majority believes that grownups are nice to them.

The next set of figures (Figures 12–16) show the response of the older youth, the ones in the Simba program. Note that baseline and follow-up data are available. Also note that the numbers seeing violent incidents are higher then for the Spirit youth. Clear majorities had seen violent episodes or illegal activities.

There are rarely personal attacks. Violence at home is rarely reported. Even violent threats are uncommon at home; unlike the reports of the Spirit youth, they report feeling safe both at home and school (Figure 13).

Like Spirit youth they feel adults are nice to them.

In virtually all figures they report similar responses in the follow-up period, showing that the results are reliable.

"Levonn" is an assessment instrument for very young children in which the child has read a series of vignettes that are accompanied by a cartoon character that the child can identify with who acts out the statement (Figure 14). This instrument was presented only to the Spirit youth to get self-perception of sadness and violent tendencies. Only a few youth endorsed statements were consistent with consequences from violent exposure.

Nevertheless, those that reported being upset were less likely to do so in the reassessment. This view was endorsed by a majority of youth but fewer youth endorsed them in the reassessment.

Clinical assessments were more meaningful for the Simba participants. Six were referred for screening and all met full DSM-II-R criteria for posttraumatic stress disorder, including flashbacks, hyperactivity, emotional blunting, and avoidant behavior. Over half of the participants reported at least one symptom. Two of the participants that met full

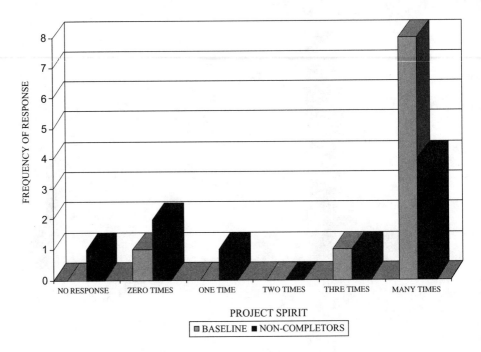

Figure 12.   Question 2: I have heard guns being shot—Project Simba.

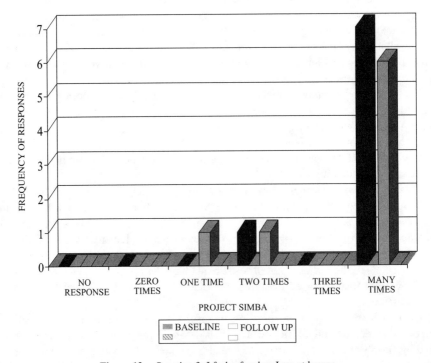

Figure 13.   Question 3: I feel safe when I am at home.

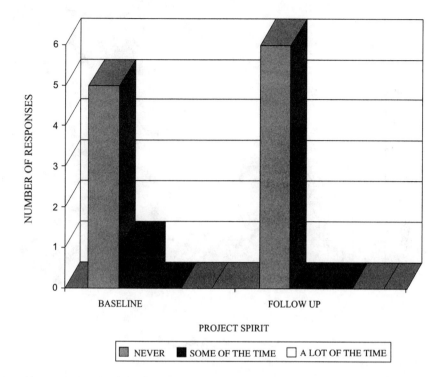

6

5

NUMBER OF RESPONSES

4

3

2

1

0

BASELINE   FOLLOW UP

PROJECT SPIRIT

☐ NEVER   ■ SOME OF THE TIME   ☐ A LOT OF THE TIME

Figure 14.   Levonn is really scared about something bad happening to him when he goes outside of his house and wants to stay at home.

criteria for PTSD had previously been diagnosed as attentional deficit hyperactivity disorder and were on stimulant medication during the school year. Those with full symptoms of PTSD were either referred or their therapist contacted. Other participants and their parents were given information about local providers.

The higher the score, the greater the African Consciousness, i.e. self-identified as Afrocentric and knowledgeable about African culture and history. Four of six Simba participants in whom data were available for both sessions showed an increase in African Consciousness.

Grade point average was also determined. Grades of the Project Spirit participants showed a substantial increase (Figure 15). It was across the board and happened with most students. The number of A's and B's almost doubled. Improvements were seen in science and math (Figure 16).

Teacher conduct ratings were also measured. "Satisfactory" or better ratings increased while "needs improvement" ratings declined.

The Simba participants showed a mixed result. Overall, grade point average actually showed a slight decline. This decline seemed to be in reading courses while math performance did not change. Behavior ratings were not available for the Simba participants but qualitative data were used. Parents most often endorsed the statement that "he does what he is supposed to do" and "the program turned him around, I was really worried." Teachers endorse similar comments and both teachers and parents perceived the students as doing better in school despite the drop in grade point average. One student, with frequent incarcerations, avoided arrest since the program began.

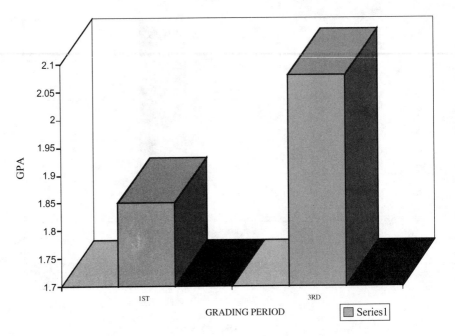

Figure 15.   Mean GPA-Spirit.

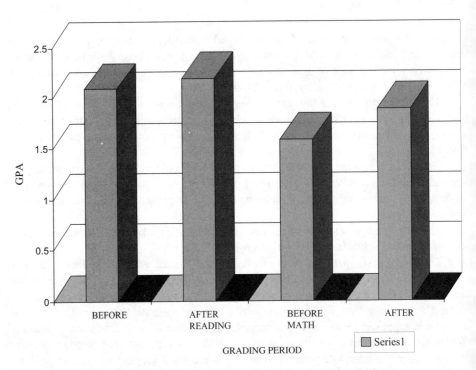

Figure 16.   Mean value GPA for reading and math—Project Spirit.

Youth commented: "I have something to do with my time, "my mother is getting along with me better" and "the program is great, I learned a lot of new things".

Discussion and Conclusions

African American male youth in an inner city area of a midsize midwestern city were enrolled in an after school enrichment and violence prevention program. Many of the students were exposed to violence as has been reported with other inner city areas (Bell & Jenkins, 1993; Osofsky et al., 1994). Consistent with those reports we noted that the violence was not a result of attacks to the youth personally or to violence exposures at home. Consistent with these reports we found that these youth felt safe at home and school. Unlike these other reports the younger participants did not feel safe at home. Perhaps older youth recognized the limitations of parent protection while the younger participants felt more dependent on their parents and perhaps blamed them for failing to protect them from the community violence.

The violence was ever-present in the community. Consistent with other reports the quality of the violence was consistent with these youth living in a "battle zone" (Bell and Jenkins, 1991; Lorion and Saltzman, 1993). The reliability of the response suggested that the degree of violence in the community did not change during the time of the program. Exposure seemed to be ongoing and constant.

References

Bell, C.C. & Jenkins, E.J. *Traumatic stress and children*. Journal of Health for the poor and underserved, 1991; 2:175–185.

Bell, C.C. & Jenkins, E.J. Community violence and children on Chicago's Southside. *Psychiatry*, 1993; 56:46–54.

Deblinger, E., McLeer, S.V. Atkins, M.S., & Foa, E. Posttraumatic stress disorder in sexually abused, physically abused, and non-abused children. *Child Abuse and Neglect*. 1989; 13:403–408.

Dubrow N.F. & Gabarino, J. Living in the war zone: mothers and young children in public housing development. *Journal of Child Welfare*. 1989; 68:3–20.

Durant, R.H., Cadenhead, C., Pendergast, R.A., Slavens, C., & Linder, C.W. Factors associated with the use of violence among urban black adolescents. *American Journal of Public Health*. 1994; 84:612–617.

Famularo, R., Kinscharff, R., & Fenton, T. Symptom differences in acute and chronic presentation of childhood posttraumatic stress disorder. *Child Abuse and Neglect*. 1990; 14:439–444.

Freeman, L.M., Mokros, H., & Poznanski E.O. Violent events reported by urban school aged children: characteristics and depression correlates. *Journal of the American Academy of Child and Adolescent Psychiatry*. 1993; 32:419–423.

Garbarino, J., Kostelyn, K., & Dubrow, N. No place to be a child: Growing up in a war zone. *Lexington Books*, 1991.

Griffith, E.H. & Bell, C.C. Recent trends in suicide and homicide among blacks. *Journal of the National Medical Association*. 1989; 262:2265–2269.

Kiser, L.J., Heston, J., Millsap. P.A.A., & Pruitt, D.B, Physical and sexual abuse in childhood: relationship with post-traumatic stress disorder. *Journal of the American Academy and Child arid Adolescent Psychiatry*. 1991; 30:776–783.

Lawson, W.B. *Psychiatric diagnosis of African Americans in: Cross cultural psychiatry*. Edited by Herrera J.M. Lawson, WB. Starnek, J.J. Chichestere Wiley, 1999.

Lorion, R.P. & Saltzman, W. Children's exposure to community violence: following a path from concern to research to action. *Psychiatry*. 1993; 56:55–65.

Maras, S. & Cohen, D. *Children and inner-city violence; strategies for intervention.*

Leavift, L. & N. Fox (Eds.). *Psychological effects of war and violence on children*. Hillsdale, NJ: Eribaum, 1993; pp. 281–302.

McLeer, S.V. Deblinger, E., Atkins, M.S., Foa, R.B., & Ralphe, D.L. Posttraumatic stress disorder in sexually abused children. *Journal of the American Academy of Child and Adolescent Psychiatry*. 1988; 27:650–654.

Osofsky, J.D. The effects of exposure to violence on young children. *American Psychologist*. IM; 782–788.

Pynoos, R.S. & Nader, K. Psychological first aid and treatment approaches to children exposed to community violence: research implications. *Journal of Traumatic Stress*. 1988; 1:445–73.

Pynoos, R.S. & Eth, S. Developmental perspectives on psychic trauma in childhood. In R.C. Figley (Ed.). *Trauma and its wake*. New York: Brunner/Mazel. 1985.

Pynoos, R.S. Traumatic stress and developmental psychopathology in children and adolescents. In J.M. Oldham, M.B. Riba & A. Tasman (Eds.). *American Psychiatric Press review of psychiatry* (Vol. 12). Washington, DC; American Psychiatric Press. 1993.

Richters, J.E. & Martinez, P. *The NIMH community violence project*. Children as victims of and witnesses to violence. *Psychiatry*. 1993; Vol. 1, 56:7–21.

Rosenberg, M.L., O'Carrol, P.W., & Powell, K.E. Lets be clear; violence is a public health problem. *Journal of the American Medical Association*. 1992; 267:3071–3072.

Runyan, C.W. & Gerken, E.A. Epidemiology and prevention of adolescent injury, a review and research agenda. *Journal of the American Medical Association*. 1989; 262:2273–2279.

Shakoor, B.H. & Chalmers, D. Co-victimization of African-American children who witness violence: Effects on cognitive, emotional, and behavioral development. *Journal of the National Medical Association*. 1991; 83:233–237.

6

Applying Mental Health Behavioral Change to Ethnonational Conflict Resolution

MAURICE APPREY

The Health Behavioral Change Imperative and the Clinician

This chapter takes the position that clinical practitioners who carry out interventions under the rubric of *Health Behavioral Change Imperative* need *a wide range of clinical skills.* Although this approach to behavioral change takes the community as a primary target rather than the individual for change, it is inevitable that clinical practitioners would at various times meet situations that require them to have skills for intervention with individuals, families, youth groups, gangs, and teenage pregnancy groups, among other target populations.

Secondly, with the collapse of nation states like the Soviet Union, nationalism is on the rise and increasingly, the psychology of neighbors with ethnic strife between them cries out for containment and transformation. *Clinical practitioners, at home and abroad, therefore, need to have tools for solving ethnic conflicts.*

Thirdly, to the extent that the health behavioral change imperative requires the clinician to implement change from the standpoint of the community, clinicians need to know the *history of the communities that they wish to change.* For example, clinicians need to know what kind of vibrant community it was before a major highway was constructed straight through or around that community causing it to be split or isolated. What did the highway do to the sewer system? Did it ensure that the sewer system of the rich was now separated from that of the poor? Did the city planners ensure that the public transport system was now in one place where it did not connect the poorer community to the industry that would hire workers? Before the highway, was it the case that every morning people woke up to the smell of tobacco, reminding them that it was time to go to work? Now, thanks to the highway, the public may wake up to the smell of broken sewer lines.

Clinicians, then, must know the layout of the community and the history behind it. In addition to the ecological history, they must know the cultural history of the community. In a previous work (Apprey, 1999) it was noted that communities who have historically been victims of racism and oppression are constantly on an errand. Individuals, families and communities that are most successful in transforming themselves find *new ways to improve their condition by extricating themselves from the original transgressor's errand to reduce them to nothing*, in the case of African-Americans; or, to ashes, in the case of people of Jewish origins. In contrast, practitioners of Black-on-Black crime have lost sight of the original enemy and the errand to be nothing or dead.

Transgressed groups, then, are threatened by *urgent, voluntary, errands*. What is *urgent* is that they peremptorily find ways to destroy themselves according to their original transgressor's wishes. What is *voluntary* is that they choose their own poison. Successful communities, then, must find new and ethical ways to renew or transform themselves.

Unfortunately, the psychological toxin of self-destruction injected by the likes of Willy Lynch and his kind can also run in families from generation to generation. As a result, multiple versions of self-destruction plague transgressed groups. It is therefore incumbent on clinicians that they take an ecological history, a cultural history, as well as take time to know the families or groups within the community who are most affected by the oppressive history.

A health behavioral imperative, therefore, requires clinical practitioners to study how a community takes the events of history and turns them into a sense of history, thereby storing in various ways the errand of destruction. In this respect, clinicians must understand how poor eating habits with destructive consequences can be part of the errand toward a community's extinction. Heart attacks, diabetes, and other medical conditions are all implicated in how oppressed communities have appropriated the psychological toxins of history.

---

1. The events of history can be changed to a sense of history
2. Sedimentations of history are activated in present contexts and then extended to deal with contemporary issues.
3. Cultural memory is the means of defining a group's experience of trauma and the strategy for storing and deferring the traumatic infusion by the transgressor.
4. Ethnonational and intercultural conflicts can be reworked in the relatively safe and contained setting of conflict resolution work or nation-building programs conducted by third party facilitators. The conceptual basic assumptions that subserve the conduct and management of ethnonational conflict resolution serve as anchor for third party facilitators. They are reminders that the work of conflict resolution depends on process and must not be precipitously foreclosed into structured or fixed ideas.
5. The process of working in small groups with influential people from both parties is essential in the promotion of dialogue, which in turn transforms psychological experience when there is appropriate third party facilitation. Out of these intense, small working groups will come conflict management projects that include activities at local sites.
6. Two contrasting local projects are briefly described.

Figure 17.   Trajectory of issues for consideration regarding ethnonational conflict resolution.

This chapter is a careful attempt to provide the theoretical underpinnings behind practices of community intervention. In this author's view, when clinicians know why they do what they do, they are more likely to practice with more confidence and with decisively more effective interventions. Consistent with the view that clinical practitioners must have skills that work at home and abroad, this chapter provides a relatively generic theoretical frame of reference and ends with a case example from Eastern Europe.

Introducing Transgenerational Haunting and the Pivot of Difference and Identity

Manifestations of violent ethnonational conflicts are inseparable from history. Invariably, these forms of conflict are subserved by the shift *from events of history to a contemporary sense of history*. In this respect we are dealing with *appropriations of history*. The psychoanalyst Heinz Hartmann (1958) spoke to this issue of appropriation in ways that are consistent with my understanding of historical transformations:

> Man does not come to terms with his environment anew in every generation; his relation to the environment is guaranteed by an evolution peculiar to man, namely, the influence of tradition and the survival of the works of man. *We take over from others a great many of our methods for solving problems*. The works of man objectify the methods he has discovered from solving problems and thereby become factors of continuity, so that *man lives*, so to speak, in *past generations as well as in his own*. (p. 30; emphasis added.)

In addition to the transgenerational transmission of destructive aggression, the appropriations of history have very specific contents. With respect to violent ethnonational conflicts, the pivotal issues are *difference and identity*. It is as if humans had an obligation, albeit self-imposed, to cleanse and purify ourselves, in order to purge ourselves of some inchoate and unmetabolized parts of ourselves. These parts of ourselves which we dare not admit as belonging to us must therefore be housed elsewhere; or worse, deposited to the world of *no place*, namely, death of the Other. Introducing transgenerational haunting and difference/identity, the transgenerational serves as the vertical axis and issues of difference and identity as occupying the place of the horizontal axis. Within the realm of the vertical, there lie the static events of history. Within the realm of the horizontal, there lies the modern day drama of turning the events of history into lived experience.

Before spelling out precisely how humans live in the past as well as in the present and what they do with the Other to purify themselves and to render the Other inferior, useless, or dead, it is useful to plot a trajectory of how the events of history become appropriated as a sense of history, a process of *staging*.

Staging and Transforming Historical Grievances: The Sedimentation and Reactivation of Cultural Memory

The Estonian semiotician Yurij Lotman and his co-worker B.A. Uspensky (1971) defined culture as "the nonhereditary memory of a community, a memory expressing itself in a system of constraints and prescriptions" (p. 411). Treating culture as a social phenomenon and specifically as a memory and record of what a community has experienced, they connected culture to past historical experience. Culture then "is only perceived ex post facto" (p. 411). To be precise, "When people speak of the creation of a new culture, they are inevitably looking ahead; that is, they have in mind that which they presume will become a memory from the point of view of the reconstructable future" (p. 412).

In his *Cartesian Meditations*, the German philosopher Edmund Husserl (1929) wrote of the dialectic between sedimentation (fading) and reactivation (recall) and the strategy of reducing historical fact to a sense of and a reconstitution of that historical fact. Ernesto Laclau (1990), an Argentinian political scientist, echoing Husserl, wrote on the shift from historical givens to *new conditions of possibility*. Along similar lines, the German literary theorist Wolfgang Iser (1992) built on the work of the later Husserl to articulate his notion of staging as lived anthropological category rather than as a reflected epistemological category. Staging, for Iser, "must always be preceded by something to which it has to give appearance" (p. 885).

He continues:

> This 'something' can never be completely covered by the staging, because otherwise staging itself would become its own enactment. In other words, every staging lives in what it is not. For everything that materialized in it stands in the service of something absent, which, although given presence through something else that is present, cannot be present itself. Staging is thus an absolute form of doubling, not least because it always retains awareness that this doubling is ineradicable (p. 885).

What enables staging, according to Iser, to make such a separation between an historical given and its new presentation is its inherent separation between the historical mode and the new something that is to be given appearance. Staging, then, encompasses past and present, absence and concrete presentation, a given and a simulacrum, fading and recall, as well as extension and supplementation of that which is being reactivated and recalled.

This journey from cultural memory through recall to transformation of historical grievances and how this journey is operationalized into praxis is the subject of this chapter.

Some Specific Modes of Storage of Cultural Memory: Anticipating Praxis

In order to overturn destructive appropriations of history, a heuristic approach for unmasking originary but persistent mandates must be undertaken. The heuristic approach refers to experimental and pre-theoretical ideas that can be tested in the field, given up if they do not work, and stabilized into theory if they can be shown to merit serious consideration. Originary *and persistent mandates*, refer to the mandate to preserve the originary legacy of ashes in new, but equally destructive, forms. It is as if the motor of destruction remains but the license plate changes.

The psychoanalytic notion of *change of function*, according to Hartmann (1958) suggests, "What defensive operations were anchored in instincts may subsequently be performed in the service of and by means of the ego, though naturally, new regulations too will arise in the course of development of the ego and the id" (p. 49). He continues: "Differentiation progresses not only by creation of new apparatuses to master new demands and new tasks, but also and mainly by new apparatuses taking over, on a higher level, functions which were performed by more primitive means" (p. 50).

Change of function can manifest itself in destructive ways, such as murder in one generation, suicide in the next. Or, it can manifest itself in a higher form when the next generation chooses a more productive means of survival. Four specific means of rupture and storage of cultural memory shall be considered. Appropriating Hillis Miller (1992), a four-step heuristic strategy is suggested (see Apprey, 1999) to observe and ultimately transform received hatred from an Other group. These four rubrics are related, but they are separated here in order to effect greater clarity. The key rubrics of the heuristic strategy are: (1) line, (2) character, (3) anastamosis, that is transgenerational haunting, and (4) figure.

Under the rubric of line, we may think of a broken line, a cut, an incision, a gap, rupture, lost ancestry as in the wound of an absence in the African American lineage. Into this cut, may be inserted a world of lived experience where the oppressed have lost sight of the original enemy and may attack their own, as in *Black-on-Black* crime, or variants of lost identity.

Under the rubric of character (from the Greek word kharassein, "to brand") we may think of a scratch into the skin, the verbs to engrave, to make a deep impression, to carve; in short, to put a hot rod in blazing fire, make a deep branding impression on the skin of a slave, and in so branding him or her, declare the signification "I own you." Or, a Nazi soldier may pin a Star of David on the chest of a Jewish person and declare the constructed signification, "You are vermin. You must burn."

These two ideas, line and character, can be examined together. The cut into a line introduces a rupture in the identity of a people, creating a potential hole in their world. However, the branding, which once existed in the original mandate of slavery, can now change from one hand to another. A reversal of agency can now occur both in the world of the broken line, or, in the means of preserving the poisonous history. Witness excessive use of tattoos or hair coloring as modes of preserving the poison of reversal of agency. Horizonal with the words, "broken line" and "character" are two terms used by the French psychoanalyst, Jean Laplanche (1999) "intromission" and "implantation." He uses these terms with respect to individual pathological formations. However, they will serve the description of shared injury to and branding of a people. Laplanche (1999) writes, "implantation is a process which is common, everyday, normal or neurotic" (p. 136). But it has a virulent variant, which can be invoked here, Laplanche (1999) writes:

> Besides it [that is, apart from the normal or neurotic], as its violent variant, a place must be given to *intromission*. While implantation allows the individual to take things up actively, at once translating and repressing, one must try to conceive of a process which blocks this, short-circuits the differentiation of the agencies in the process of their formation, and puts into the interior an element resistant to all metabolization (p.136).

According to Laplanche, then, "implantation allows the injured party to actively take things up, as well as attempt to translate or repress the injury. Intromission, however, forecloses translation or transformation. Instead, it renders the injury resistant to change. Laplanche's words are worth repeating: intromission short-circuits differentiation and puts into the interior an element resistant to all metabolization" (p. 136). Using the body and its skin-envelope as well as the orifices of the body as metaphor, Laplanche (1999) writes: "Intromission relates principally to anality and orality. Implantation refers, rather, to the surface of the body as a whole, its perceptive periphery" (p. 137).

Laplanche's distinction is that the skin remembers (implantation) when it is broken into, whether it is a matter of a subject seeing and/or remembering a massacre of people, or a subject concretely and actively receiving pain from torture. I imagine further from Laplanche's description that sodomy (intromission via anality) is known by perpetrators of ethnic violence as the most shaming strategy. In the United States, the case of white

New York City policemen forcibly inserting a toilet plunger into a black man's anus and mouth speaks amply to this issue of intromission as a shaming strategy. Laplanche does not mention intromission via the genitals, but we can add it to the repertoire of shaming devices when perpetrators of ethnic violence rape the mothers, wives, and daughters of the enemy. For the male relatives of these assaulted women, it is as if they themselves have been raped and sodomized. For them, it is a vicarious homosexual assault not easily forgotten or transformed. In Laplanche's language, these strategies of intromission cause injuries that are not easily metabolized.

Carolivia Herron's (1991) description of generations of African Americans suffering the vicissitudes of transgenerational trauma demonstrates the rubric of transgenerational haunting. Below is a summary:

1. The females shall be raped by slave masters; the males shaft be murdered by slave masters.
2. The males who are not murdered shall be sold away.
3. The males who are neither murdered nor sold away shall marry females who are not murdered or sold away.
4. In marriage, enslaved males and former slaves shall have revenge over females perceived to have consented to the destruction of males.
5. Women and daughters shall therefore be raped over and over again by enslaved men or former slaves.

This is a sequence of appropriative and appositional shifts and transfers where there occurs (1) the historical presentation of rape and murder in the first instance; (2) appropriation by an ethnic group of a transgressor's cruelty, to serve a secondary purpose of revenge; and (3) ossification of a structure of experience that says that victims may heap cruelty that once originated with external transgressors onto their own kind.

In transgenerational haunting, then, a concrete staging, a doubling, a reactivation of sedimented historical grievances, a replay and an extension occur, and it is this transformation that starts this process of losing sight of one's historical enemies.

Finally, under the rubric of figure, we may think of a torturer disfiguring the Other; a colonizer reducing a human being's status from a citizen to a *non*-person, a slave owner in the American South reducing a human being to 3/5 of a person, and from the historical instance of exchange of goods (metaphor) to the perverse metonymy of selling persons as in slavery. Dehumanization, par excellence, subserves this rubric.

I have so far considered history as that which is reconstituted by groups in conflict. Sedimentations of historical grievances are reactivated and then extended by those who choose to relive them. In observing aggrieved people, we have an obligation to know the actual historical injury, how it is mentalized and extended. We have a further obligation to understand the historical motivation behind acts of aggression such as the mandate to render an Other group extinct, or an errand to render an Other group slaves or dead. Knowing the mandate or errand will subsequently tell us how the aggrieved group has stored the historical memory. We would need to know what the aggrieved group has stored in that imaginary space of a broken line; what reversal of agency has taken place so that they are harming their own by their own hand, having lost sight of the original enemy. We would need to know the many ways in which traumatic history has been deferred, and to what extent the aggrieved group has been disfigured, dehumanized and remains traumatized as a people.

From the transgressor's end, the question still needs to be asked: How does the transgressor group store its cultural memory? Owing to space limitations, listed below is what might be considered to be the central strategy: (1) the power to define socio-economic, political and even psychological issues in a community; (2) the power to write history and to publish according to the claims of the group that has greater power; (3) the power to disseminate that history and (4) the power to define how that history is taught in schools. For example, when American children are taught only U.S. history from 1800 onward, a psychological statement is made to the children: that they may obliterate prior African and European history, or that they may define themselves in terms of the power relations between minority and majority groups.

Given how crucial it is to grasp the vicissitudes of cultural memory, it becomes essential that during the conflict resolution process feuding parties are given opportunities to engage in an on-going process where history can be staged, relived and worked through.

Praxis: Heuristic Steps for Negotiating Ethnonational Conflicts: The Case of Estonia and Its Russians

The Center for the Study of Mind and Human Interaction (CSMHI) of the University of Virginia School of Medicine is an interdisciplinary center whose work in conflict resolution requires the collaboration of psychoanalysts, historians, diplomats and other scholars. Over the past decade, CSMHI has been invited to participate in the resolution of conflicts between nations as well as other related ethnonational and factional disputes.

Following the breakup of the Soviet Union, Estonia wished to restore its political, as well as its psychological, independence. CSMHI had participated in other cases with participants from both 'Russia and Estonia, and accordingly, became an excellent and credible candidate to assist both sides in the process of Estonia's psychopolitical independence from Russia, and co-existence with Russia as its neighbor. The methods of CSMHI have been described elsewhere. One description of the group's methods (see Apprey, 1996) posits four heuristic steps in the conflict resolution process, which are meant to be suggestive, but not exhaustive or cast in stone. Briefly then, the following constitute the steps in the operations of CSMHI:

1. Intensive confidential interviews are conducted with a cross-section of leaders from all constituencies to ensure that CSMHI personnel understand the historical and contemporary concerns facing Estonians, and Russians who have chosen to live in Estonia after the collapse of the Soviet Union.

2. A series of psychopolitical dialogues between representatives of interested parties (20–30 in large, plenary sessions, to open and close each day of talks, and 8–10 people in small work group sessions). During these dialogues, lines of communication are opened, concerns shared and hidden psychological barriers that divide interested parties are brought to the surface, discussed, and ultimately transformed, so that they no longer impede negotiation and movement toward common goals. The process often involves recognizing the influence of historical relationships and events, how they recur, and how they change function when they are perpetuated under different guises to serve new purposes. This second step is essential to the success of step three.

3. Cooperative development of, or investment in, specific strategies and projects based on the new understanding of the divisive issues that have surfaced during the

dialogues. Projects emerge from psychopolitical dialogue, based on newly-established coalitions between members, their shared needs, and the sense that the implementation of these projects is going to be part of a longer term process of change. In this third step, the parties in conflict undertake projects jointly, and they do so with *input* from the third party facilitators.

4. The third party (CSMHI) withdraws as the community continues working toward common goals, through dialogues that complement and support ongoing projects. Thus, the fourth step involves projects independently undertaken by the groups hitherto in conflict but *without input* from the third party facilitators.

What Happens in the Psychopolitical Dialogue?

The section below explores in some detail the dialogue in the second way station of the methodology. When one works in small groups with two parities in conflict, the group work typically begins with polarization as the first step.

Polarization

Under the category of polarization the Other is demonized. The Other is imagined to be a terrible Other. That Other has a marginal status. Preconstructed as dangerous, the Other is posited in close juxtaposition to the subject's own relatively favored position.

Differentiation within Each Faction

Under the rubric of differentiation within each integral faction (or selfsame subject system) a second phase follows when facilitators have permitted the process of polarization to take place, and have allowed it to assume the necessary function of self-definition and clarification of borders between the two sides.

Here, differentiation within each side becomes possible because of the emerging recognition of paradoxes within the ideological positions of each faction. Here, as de Certeau (1984), Dollimore (1991), and Uebel (1996) indicate, the border between participants of each faction are recognized as having a double status as marker of separation, and a line of commonality within each side. In this respect "to be against," that is, "opposed to, is also to be against, that is, close up, in proximity to, or, in other words, up against." (Dollimore, 1991, p. 229). For example, when Estonians fight for Soviets against Estonians, who fight for Nazis, they are against each other, or opposed to each other. Yet because both sides are Estonians they are close to each other or proximal to each other. In short they are both close to and up against each other.

The Threshold of Border Crossing and the Crossing of Mental Borders

In this third way-station of the two sides negotiating and subsequently crossing mental borders, both sides encounter together the trauma and obsession of their historical grievances. Here, the place and function of dialogue as that which create mental spaces, which open up new illusionistic spaces, present themselves. Borderlines open up and become recognized as potential spaces between the two disputing factions.

These gaps, or middle spaces, which have now become illusionistic spaces for bridge building (Pruyser, 1983), now symbolize exchange and encounter that facilitate an eventual crossing of mental borders. This crossing of mental borders effects the transformation of the trauma and obsession of historical grievances. This third way station is preeminently a place of playfulness and fantastic metaphorization of conflicting positions admixed with serious dialogue. For example, an observer might hear something like: "When you love a woman, you must say it often enough so that she'd believe you."

This crossing of mental borders that transforms trauma and obsession of historical grievances operates so that the two sides that had been polarized now operate conjunctly. Here, one term proposes the other for its meaning. The hitherto absolutely Other is integrated to the self same subject system through encounter with and resolution of ambivalence. In making complementarities out of antinomies, absence or exclusion simultaneously become a presence. It is not until this way station reaches a peak of metaphorization, with both sides contributing to the new imagery and imagining, that the establishment of common ground can be trusted.

The Establishment of Common Ethical Positions and/or Pragmatic Solutions

In this final way station of the creation of new and adaptive solutions, ethical positions and trial actions of mutual responsibility emerge. These ethical positions lead to pragmatic projects as indices of internalization of new and generalizable adaptive solutions.

Community Projects

Earlier it was mentioned that in the overall method of the conflict resolution program there is the sequence of (1) the diagnostic phase (assessment), (2) the psychopolitical process (dialogue), (3) projects conducted by the feuding groups with the assistance of the third party facilitators, and (4) projects without the third party facilitators. Without the fourth step, the ability to assess the success of the third-party facilitators would be limited. A successful fourth step, then, would indicate sustainability of the original project by the community, and its capacity to generalize outcomes into other communities that need interethnic conflict resolution programs.

Below are very brief accounts of two community projects that were undertaken by CSMHI from 1997 to 1999. These two examples stand in sharp contrast to each other, and yet each project has legitimacy.

Selection of Sites and Rationale. Each site must have approximately 50% of indigenous Estonian speakers and 50% Russian speakers.

With this numerical parity, each project site is assisted by the facilitators to (1) form a non-governmental organization (NGO) to undertake the practical tasks involved in community building; (2) decide in a democratic fashion and through a process of dialogue how they would spend $50,000 USD to create a mutually acceptable project.

In the first year (1997–1998) they meet weekly, biweekly, or monthly, and by the end of the year should have a consensus. In the second year (1998–1999) they implement their chosen project. The decision-making process is the most crucial exercise in creating a civic democratic process. Whereas decisions generally came from Moscow during the Soviet period, these groups must now practice decision making in a democratic way on their own.

The psychological component of the dialogue process cannot be underestimated. Without it, the groups might precipitously choose a project and still hate each other, therefore, limiting the full impact of the integration project, and possibly resulting in the opposing sides sabotaging each other.

Project Hand-in-Hand at Mustamåe.   Mustamåe, a suburb of Tallinn, is the location for multiple kindergarten sites which are segregated according to language, Estonian or Russian. The kindergarten age in Estonia is 2 1/2 to 6 years of age. It is a popular notion for indigenous Estonians to think of Russian children as more boisterous, and that if the two groups of children were to be educated together in the same kindergarten, the Russians would run over the Estonians. By policy, the ratio of Russian to Estonian children who are educated in Estonian kindergartens is 1 : 5.

From the point of view of a child analyst, the perceptions of children that end up in policy are significant. A visit to Russian kindergartens and Estonian kindergartens to get a sense of each one of them before the project begins helps deepen one's understanding. Russian children are relatively active in showing their enjoyment of the creative arts, whereas their Estonian counterparts are relatively sedentary. But the difference is neither remarkable, nor attributable to some vice in one group. Both groups were interested in cowboys and Indians in our global world. It has been noted that the Estonian government wants Russian residents of Estonia to learn the Estonian language in order to become full citizens. There exists a potential situation where there would be anxiety about Russians knowing the Estonian language, because knowing a language also paves a way to knowing how to predict the world of the Other. Therefore, it is necessary to treat this project with every deliberate discretion. Although high-level members of the Estonian government asked for this project long before the NGO chose it, one may not assume that there would be no resistance to it. Therefore, there would be limited publicity at the beginning.

The Mustamåe Project, Hand-in-Hand, was a two-tiered project: the first part being the teaching of the Estonian language to 240 Russian children in 14 Russian kindergartens. The second part is an interactional one where the Russian children communicate in Estonian language to Estonian children, play with them, sing with them, undertake mutually beneficial projects, etc.

The criteria for success were established by an independent evaluator, Jay Rothman (1997) Figure 18.

All these criteria for success were met.

1. A new model for teaching Estonian language to young Russians was created. Two editions of a textbook and a teacher's edition were written for the project, and for the first time in Estonia, by the head of the NGO, Ly Krikk.

2. A governmental foundation charged with funding integration projects funded the project after CSMHI completed their work, demonstrating ownership for the project by the government.

3. There is a broader community impact in language education. Russian parents, too, now have classes to learn the language themselves. There is now a new-found three tier integration effort taking place: 'Russian parents now interact with Estonian parents, Estonian children interact with Russian children more than ever, Russian teachers and Estonian teachers now have on-going and joint continuing education activities to ensure that the development of Russian and Estonian children remains a human issue rather than exclusively a Russian issue or Estonian issue. The 1 to 5 Russian-to-Estonian classroom

Criteria for success	Measures/Indicators of criteria
1. Establish model for teaching Estonian language to Russian kindergarten children.	• Help group use their knowledge and experience to create an effective program; • Select language teachers for project by group in August; • Help children in Mustamåe with integration; • Consult with pedagogical scholars and education and cultural ministries to create effective programs.
2. Create a way to continue program after one year of funding is over.	• Group will identify new funding sources for the future; • Political allies from education ministry will be cultivated; • The project will continue past when CSMHI (PEW) money ends.
3. Broader community impact in Mustamåe (beyond language education program).	• Activities of group/NGO will be diversified (more than just a language program); • NGO will provide vehicle for discussion; • NGO will provide vehicle for discussion of broader community issues—forums and dialogues will take place; • Parents and teachers involved in NGO will educate the rest of the community about the need to integrate Russian and Estonian children.
4. Organized community group that continues work after CSMHI departure	• Group will be officially registered as NGO; • New members will be included in the NGO; • A conceptual focus will evolve instead of a technical focus—i.e. dialogue processes rather than a specific language project; • The NGO will decide its own future direction and future projects.
5. CSMHI will be an intellectual consultant to group's work and project.	• CSMHI will provide lectures and intellectual resources on child development, parent education; • CSMHI will continue to provide connections to scholarly support of NGO's work.

Figure 18.   Mustamåe.

ratio has now changed in many of the Estonian kindergartens. The language teachers employed by the NGO are now being integrated into the regular educational system. The children of the Hand-in-Hand project are now vigorously sought after by elementary schools one year ahead of time.

4. The NGO and its teachers are continuing with their work after the CSMHI pullout.

5. However, we remain consultants to teachers, scholars, and high-level government officials to advance their integration efforts. The government is even in a position to show-case its efforts toward integration of its Russian citizens in their desire to become part of the European Union and NATO.

These results reflect the need to vigilantly understand history, how it is sedimented, reactivated and extended, as well as how a praxis for a conflict resolution process takes into account polarization of views by feuding parties as a starting point in the process of dialogue. The process continues with the multiplicity of views within each faction, fol-lowed by the crossing of mental borders and finally concludes with the establishment of an ethic of responsibility. It is this ethic of responsibility that gets operationalized when feuding parties choose to carry out community projects together. Finally, the facilitators must know how to end the formal part of their involvement, and how to transition their efforts into offering consultations when they are requested.

Klooga Project: "Klooga, Our Home"

A second example of projects in the third phase of the conflict resolution process comes from the Klooga community in Estonia. This brief account demonstrates the transforma-tion of cultural memory. A detailed account of this process at Klooga has been given else-where (see Apprey, 1998). Here, as in Mustamåe, Klooga must form an NGO. They, too, have $50,000 USD to spend in the effort. In order to facilitate their democratic decision-making, the US facilitators had to begin a psychological process within this group of 20 NGO members. Later the NGO established its own criteria for expanding the member-ship in this group in order to enable it to become a larger community organization. They do this to dispel the notion that they are an exclusive club with American money to bum.

Klooga was once a concentration camp site for the Nazis. Here there are some two thousand victims buried in a mass grave. Klooga later became a Soviet military camp. Upon restoration of independence, Klooga became an Estonian military site where joint Baltic, NATO and other military exercises take place.

Klooga then, is a site where a *change of function* has taken place. It used to be a place for killing victims of the Nazis. It became a place for preparing to kill or exile Estonians. Now Klooga is a place for reminding the Russians who live there that the town is etched in the cultural memory of Estonia, that it is still perceived to be a dangerous place. Accordingly, there are periodic incidents of shooting during military exercises which the citizens' find rather disruptive to their daily lives.

Because there is a psychological process, a theme runs through their meetings. It is a historical reality that after independence had been restored in Estonia, the Russian military personnel returned to Russia. However, they left behind wives and children. Estonians who now live there are mostly those who came to Klooga for cheaper housing.

In the group process, the theme of dirt in Klooga is an abiding one. Klooga must be cleaned, literally. Heat must be restored. An infrastructure of law and order must be cre-ated. Issues of survival are therefore first and foremost on their minds.

After a year of dialogue between the members of the NGO, they decide to clean up and rebuild an old house donated by the county government. The NGO will now transform this building into a community center where they will hold their regular meetings and strive to become a political force. Here too, they will hold dance classes for the children, language classes for the adults and so on. Now the Klooga project will be named "Klooga: Our Home."

In the second year of the project, they organize and complete the refurbishing of the community center. There are periodic conflicts between them as they work together. For example, an Estonian man with carpentry skills feels that the women are taking over the NGO and he will not tolerate a situation where women in leadership positions do nothing but "chat about nothing." Fortunately, an Estonian psychologist on site helps them work through the problem, reframing problems and making members aware of how ethnic problems become attached to contemporary family life situations. It is important that the psychological conflicts that occur between the members of the NGO be transformed. Otherwise, it would be difficult for the participants to work together.

Consider, then, a situation where a Russian social worker is thanking an Estonian man in the group for providing hand-on services to the senior citizens with whom she works. She looks away while she talks to him about an issue, which is of tremendous value to her. When this occurrence is explored with the group, the social worker confides: "I cannot look at him because he has a very jealous wife." Personal issues, ethnic issues, familial issues, community building issues often get condensed, and it becomes the task of the facilitators to sort them out with the NGO so that the work of community building can proceed.

The criteria for success established by the independent evaluator (Figure 19, Rothman, 1997) were as follows:

One year after the building of the community center, that is, two years after the dialogue between Estonian and Russian speakers began; all criteria for success were met. The description below highlights only a few.

1. The NGO officially became registered as a tax-exempt civic organization.

2. The NGO became the infrastructure for community activities, evolving from a small group of twenty concerned citizens to one open to the entire community. Now they organize community activities with the assistance of the larger community and to the benefit of all.

3. Specifically, the community center is a site for learning activities and for civic action, a symbol of democracy.

4. The NGO members are now aware of the history of Klooga, thanks to ongoing psychological processes facilitated by the project, and a psychologically sensitive film made by the renowned Canadian filmmaker, Allan King, called "The Dragon's Eggs."

5. The process of dialogue is now an established part of decision-making in Klooga. It has replaced waiting for orders from Moscow, or waiting for the Estonian government in Tallinn to act, or waiting for their county government to meet citizens' needs.

6. One member of the NGO has completed a gathering of signatures to protest the disruptive and loud shots heard almost everyday from the military range.

7. The head of the NGO ran for political office and lost, and is running again for another political office.

8. The NGO is now poised to seek additional funds from the Estonian government for their community activities. In the meantime, members can raise more money through Estonian language lessons, bake sales, fun fairs, etc.

Each community project is unique in how it comes into its own and acquires its distinctive mark. In Mustamåe, the language teaching was part of a hot national debate. Therefore, ethnic conflicts in the NGO group dialogues were palpable from the very beginning. Russians feared that being forced to learn the Estonian language constituted a

Criteria for Success	Measure/Indicators of Criteria
1. Amplify presence and activities of NGO "Klooga: Our Home" in the community	• Settle on and secure house for community center. • Hire a director for the center. • Offer more community activities.
2. For Klooga to become a more symbolic expression of community—i.e. represent and illustrate diverse individuals working together for the good of the whole community	• Demonstrate group responsibility for community (through renovation projects, clean-up projects and general "looking out" for property). • Help Russians become Estonian citizens through language assistance. • Involve others in NGO—more members.
3. CSMHI to enhance the group building process in the community and help NGO have broader impact on the community by affecting more people and offering more people and offering more activities	• CSMHI helps cultivate contacts with Estonians political leaders. • Lead focus groups on visioning for the future of the community. • NGO will offer diversifying activities CSMHI will help facilitate process.
4. Explore the psychological aspect of Klooga's History	• Assist community to write a history of Klooga with a backward and forward focus. • Explore the hidden transcripts and historical motivations that correspond to historical moments.
5. Continue dialogue process in community	• NGO uses the same methods that they used for organizing their group (e.g. collaboration, cooperation, and involvement) in their future endeavors.
6. Find a political voice for Klooga	• NGO will appeal to leaders to address community problems (e.g. the need for new roads to the post office, military testing too dose to homes).
7. Create pride and hope for the future of the Klooga community by placing the citizens in charge of their own decisions and making Klooga a nice place to live	• Klooga will look like a "pretty place". • NGO will sponsor and organize group celebrations and festivals. • The community will have clear leadership and direction from members within the community for the first time.
8. NGO will earn its own money in the future	• NGO will organize and offer Estonian language courses as an income-generating business.

Figure 19.   Klooga: Our Home.

victory dance on their grave by Estonians, and a loss of their Russian identity and heritage. On the other hand, Estonians feared that when Russians learned the Estonian language and became full partners in the democratic process, they would constitute a large political force. After all, Russians represent one-third of the population in Estonia, a country of on-and-a-half million people.

In Klooga there were issues of survival to begin with: cleaning up, having electricity to heat homes, and so on. Therefore, the ethnic issues began to show after citizens became one inseparable "family." Now one would hear the following: More Russian children use the community center than Estonian children." To this Russians would reply: "You Estonians have better chairs and tables in your classrooms." To this Estonians would say, "Russian children have better clothes."

Ethnic conflict is now observable, and the NGO and the community can now be assisted to resolve these psychologically charged issues by talking them out rather than playing out their conflicts in destructive activity. Thanks to the project, conflicts which were manifest in the above examples (or in another more disturbing situation where the Estonian teacher and her Russian counterpart were literally throwing objects at each other across the hall between classrooms) can now be avoided, and confronted in the safer setting of a meaningful dialogue.

Epilogue: Some Do's and Don'ts

As indicated above, during the process of working with communities, the facilitator has to determine the ways in which a community has changed the *events of history* to an appropriated *sense of history*. This sense of history defines a group's experience of trauma and the strategy for storing and deferring the traumatic infusion by the transgressor. Further, there is a process that guides the delivery of interventions. That process is as follows:

1. diagnostic interviews try to capture both the history and the contemporary concerns of the community.
2. a series of psychopolitical dialogues allow representatives from various constituencies to be represented; a step in the process where elders, elected officials or their designates, law enforcement representatives, ministerial alliances, and so on, become part of the thinking through of history and what needs to be done today.
3. out of the dialogues emerge suggestions for projects and their implementation at the grass roots level and/or other spheres of the community.
4. a fourth step where the clinician or facilitator pulls out to enable the community to carry on with the changes that have begun and to take full ownership of the project(s).

It is very tempting for practitioners to skip the first two steps of diagnostic interviews with community members and the dialogues with high-level officials. To skip these two steps is like refusing to pay homage to one's elders. More importantly, these are the people who will support the project and take ownership of it when the clinician's work is done. Skipping these two steps, then, can have the following consequences. Suppose clinicians were working with a youth group on church property and halfway through, the deacon board objected to the changes in the participants. Suppose they objected on the manifest basis that the children left litter behind just before their meeting and that ever since 1897 they have always had their meetings on that Wednesday evening without interference. Suppose they objected more so to the changes the youth were making, such as becoming more intellectually stimulated, more self determined, etc; changes that were actually positive but made the deacons "afraid" that their otherwise submissive, depressed, or delinquent youth were becoming more focused, self-determined and with a wider repertoire of decision-making skills.

The critical point here is that if the first two steps were skipped, resistances from inside the community would show. After all, no community likes to change without fear, struggle or opposition to positive changes.

Of equal interest is the resistance shown by funding agencies to minority groups in transition. Community workers often speak of funds being cut just when positive changes are on the horizon. Community workers speak of how often their community police officers get transferred just when trust between them and the community is developing. Imagine then that practitioners have embarked on a project to reduce gang warfare but did not consider speaking beforehand with the local minister, the local police, or educators. This would be a recipe for failure that might otherwise have been avoided if the practitioners had paid homage to the appropriate community leaders.

As indicated above, when practitioners have group processes going on between two feuding parties, there is a tendency to seek common ground prematurely; because, the last thing two feuding factions want to hear is what they have in common. Emotionally, they experience the premature suggestion of common ground as an imposition; as mixing blood; as taboo, as incest. Or, they may pay lip service to common issues, precipitously arrive at a respectable solution but not follow through after the practitioner has left. This is why differences must first be appreciated and worked through before common ground is sought.

Finally, it is this author's opinion that the conceptual grounding behind practices must be known and articulated before interventions are made. Otherwise, two people from diametrically opposed positions may seem to have common ground. A case in point: Imagine a Jesse Helms agreeing with a Teddy Kennedy that teenage pregnancies must be avoided. One might suggest we not use government funding to support projects' the other might suggest we do. Both may think it is in our national interest to fund or not fund such projects. Nevertheless, what seemed like common ground at the very outset very quickly becomes only a nominal agreement. Similarly, many concepts in clinical practice may look like they have simply semantic differences.

However, when we take time to appreciate the epistemology or epistemic conversations behind the theories we are apt to see multiple worlds. In addition, when we have more understanding we probably have greater choices in how we select intervention strategies. Theory and practice are therefore continuous in this author's view.

References

Apprey, M. (1999). Reinventing the self in the face of received transgenerational hatred in the African American community. *Journal of Applied Psychoanalytic Studies*, 1, 2, 131–143.

Apprey, M. (1998). Staging and transforming historical grievances from cultural memory to a reconstructable future. *Journal for the Psychoanalysis of Culture and Society*, 3, 1, 81–89.

Apprey, M. (1997). Alterity as process in the resolution of ethnonational conflicts: The case of Estonia. *Journal for The Psychoanalysis of Culture and Society*, 2, 2, 121–128.

Apprey, M. (1996). Broken lines, public memory, absent memory: Jewish and African Americans coming to terms with racism. *Mind and Human Interaction*, 7, 3, 139–149.

Apprey, M. (1996). Heuristic steps for negotiating ethno-national conflicts: Vignettes from Estonia. *New Literary History*, 27, 2, 199–212.

DeCerteau, M. (1984). "Special Stories," *In The practice of Everyday Life*, trans. Steven Randall. Berkeley, CA: University of California Press.

Dollimore, J. (1991). *Sexual dissidence: Augustine to Wilde/Freud to Foucault*, Oxford: Clarendon.

Hartmann, H. (1958). *The ego and the problem of adaptation*, New York: International Universities Press.

Husserl, E. (1929). *Cartesian meditations: An introduction to phenomenology*, Translated by Dorian Cairus. The Hague: Martinus Nijhoff.

Iser, W. (1992). Staging as an anthropological category, *New Literary History*, 23, 4, 877–888.

Laclau, E. (1990). and New York: Verso. *New reflections in the revolution of our time*, London and New York; Verso

Laplanche, J. (1999). *Essays on otherness*. London and New York: Routledge.

Lotman, Y. & Uspensky, B.A. (1971). On the semiotic mechanism of culture. In H. Adams & L. Searle's (Eds.) *Critical Theory Since 1965*. Tallahassee: Florida State University Press and University Presses of Florida.

Miller, J.H. (1992). *Ariadne's thread: Story lines*. New Haven, CT: Yale University Press.

Pruyser, P. (1983). *The play of the imagination: Toward a psychoanalysis of culture*. New York: International Universities Press.

Rothman, J. (1997). Action evaluation and conflict resolution. In *Theory and Practice*. Unpublished paper presented at the National Conference in Peacemaking and Conflict Resolution.

Volkan, V.D. (1992). Ethnonationalistic rituals: *An introduction. Mind and Human Interaction*, 4 (1) pp. 3–19.

Chapter 7

Development of Authenticity in Public Health

A Culturecology Model as a Culture Critique

LEWIS M. KING

Introduction

> I, a man of color want only this;
> That the tool never possesses the man,
> That the exploitation of man by man cease forever;
> That it is possible to love and honor [humans]
> Wherever they might be.
>   FRANTZ FANON, *Black Skin, White Masks*, 1967

Fanon's plea for mankind has gone largely unaddressed in the fields of both medicine and public health. The tool of allopathic medicine has possessed the public health care system and fostered the continuing negation of the well being of millions. Practitioners of modern medicine are skilled at dealing with individuals and their acute conditions such as infections, viruses, and the breakdown of specific organs, but are inadequate in the face of chronic illnesses and their associated problems. According to one estimate (Rothman and Rice, 1998) chronic ailments cost $470 billion a year in direct health costs; indirectly, they cost an additional $234 billion in lost productivity from those who are disabled or die prematurely. Yet Americans continue to spend the major portion of their health care dollars on acute care, despite the overwhelming evidence that the major causes of premature death and disease are persistent chronic illnesses.

The real face of health problems in the U.S. is chronic illness (IOM, 1998). A vast collective of over 99 million Americans suffers from chronic ailments such as arthritis, diabetes, heart disease, high blood pressure, and cancer, which impose great hardship not only on the sufferer but also on their family members and the nation's health care system. Patients with chronic ailments represent 46% of those seeking medical care each year, but account for 76% of the nation's health care budget. Over 74% of persons with chronic conditions are under the age of 65 years. The strains from these largely invisible chronic illness epidemics will only expand as the population ages and those with the ailments become increasingly frail, disabled, and more vulnerable to the increasing pressures of social stress. In addition to the high incidence of chronic disease, research recognizes that at least half of all deaths before the age of 65 can be attributed to non-biological factors, and that another fifth result from environmental causes. These facts make it clear that such negative outcomes must be addressed as central issues in the future of effective disease prevention and health promotion.

Chapter Overview

The intent of the chapter is to raise a challenge in the training of new scholars being prepared for pubic health service, in a first-of-its-kind urban public health training program. The challenge for the young scholars is to reject the "obscene caricature" (Fanon, 1963) of Eurocentric models, overdetermined by the culture of supremacy and trapped in a lot of categorical thought, and try to forge a new reality. The focus of the chapter is a cultural critique of the dominant public health approach, and also on presenting an initial sketch of an alterative. Alternative approaches are not magical; they have to be worked out in community. This takes time, a commodity not afforded to African American scholars.

The underlying purpose of the entire chapter is on recasting public health in a concerted effort to guide model approaches more appropriate for the health care needs of the "co-morbid, multiple-risk factored" urban population. In the chapter the term African American is used to refer to the large masses of persons of color, of all ages and incomes, living in urban communities. The use of this label is not meant to imply a monolithic culture grouping, but rather to suggest a commonality of the urban experience (from issues of access to treatments) in relation to public health as a function of color. The chapter suggests a model more adequate to the service of humans in the community.

The Problem

Chronic illness not only accounts for the majority of illness, but also is most burdensome on urban and ethnic minority groups. African Americans, for instance, suffer disproportionately with chronic conditions such as diabetes (+14%), arthritis (+9%), high blood pressure (12%), heart disease (+7%), asthma (+5%), back ailments (+4%) and more recently HIV/AIDS (+6%). The very distribution of these illness-burdens represents the patterned responses (stressors) imposed on African Americans by social structure, including medicine's health beliefs and practices.

The social structure affects all. What is singular for African Americans is their unique pattern of exposure as a function of their color. African Americans are forced into a segregated social status best characterized as persistent negation. It is the marginalization as a function of persistent negation of the African American as a cultural being that is the fundamental problem. The health status of African Americans is influenced not only by the unique pattern of exposure to stressors, but also by the way they deal with (values and behavior) stress and life's adversities, with increasingly diminished social supports (Blazer, 1982; Cassel, 1976) in rapidly changing society. Social status, culture and behavior are all critical variables in this equation (Beatty, 1995). Many members of the African American population often are left with feelings of hopelessness, helplessness, isolation, anger, loss of control, and apathy when dealing with health care. This experience, coupled with stressors of the medical care system (e.g., African Americans are more likely to be uninsured and differently treated) and the economic system (e.g., less modernized health care system available and anticipatory anxiety related to their historic mistreatment by health care professionals, can create conditions that further exacerbate negative health. For example, the person may engage in denial of the presence of illness symptoms, or rely more on alternative or more trustworthy sources of support, such as family or church; or the person may remove the motivation for intervention altogether (Williams, 1998). The resultant disproportionate rate of illness among African Americans requires a redirection of our approaches to public health.

Over the last decade in particular, the increasing crisis in health care, spawned by escalating health care costs, has generated new public health formulations and models in an effort to expand beyond the narrow biological approaches of public health still trapped in the medical paradigm of "personal hygiene". The efforts in the United States, largely driven by the desire to reduce the costs associated with health care of the poor, have focused primarily on the study of the relationship between social/environmental structures and personality (Williams, 1990). Valuable and highly germane insights regarding the social environment, carcinogens, nutrition, and behavior, as examples, are now at least considered, if not yet fully integrated, into heath practice (Brownell, 1995; CDC, 1995; Hancock, 1999).

Health care theorists, in accepting this broader health perspective, have been pushed to develop new health promotion conceptual models that recognize the importance of community and societal levels of intervention. The inclusion of family members and natural helpers, the use of social networks and support systems, and the incorporation of the principles of social psychology, community organization, and empowerment education, are health promotion approaches that address environmental and societal factors associated with poor health status (Becker, 1998; Hahn, 1995).

The addition of these new variables in the mix, while most essential and welcome, has not resulted in any fundamental shift consistent with revolutions in science. Theoretical models addressing the challenge of the condition of African American communities have remained nested in the power of the medical paradigm. The new variables have been introduced as mere additions to the core of the public health model of personal hygiene. These additions have not resulted in any gains for African Americans. It appears that intervention protocols developed for the mainstream community, while helping that mainstream community, are less than effective for the African American community to which the problem migrates. The failure in addressing HIV/AIDS epidemic in African American urban communities is a classic recent example. The same is true for non-insulin dependent diabetes and cancer. The historical evidence suggests that the same pattern followed substance abuse and violence. In 1894, the medical journals of the time reported "a complete absence of acute alcoholism" in the black population (Hailer, 1971). Now, just over 100 years later, how is one to use public health to address the problems of substance abuse and violence? The public health paradigm dependent on medicalizing tendencies will be inadequate in addressing these conditions.

The culture of the paradigm that governs public health itself remains intact, as universal and given. This argument is similar, but broader than the one proposed by Nijuis and Van der Maesen (1994). There are three primary parameters to this cultural orientation— its ontology, its axiology and its epistemology (King and Nobles, 2000). Ontology attends to the essence of the dominant public health approach. In reality, "public" is seen as individual, singly or collectively, devoid of context, and outside of the hospital setting. The value premise (axiology) is reviewed as the absence of this construct called "disease." Disease is located in the biological system, or if unknown, in the social system, pending some genetic location, as in the case of alcoholism, obesity, and smoking. This value informs its epistemological premise; thus the search for cause is the search for individual genetic disease determinants, biological or psychological. These constructs are represented in the matrix of Figure 20.

"Public Health" then becomes the bookends to medicine. In its pure cultural representation, "public" is the "individual," "health" is on a continuum of "disease". Public health then becomes the early warning system of medicine. This notion of all disease as having genetic causes threatens to become even more cemented in the mind of the health establishment given the soon-to-be-released mapping of the human genome.

The notion of scientific credibility at the base of medicine is powerful, and particularly so when it fits into the profit motive of the insurance industry. Power dies hard, particularly one based on authority and control. This scientific rationalism behind the scene of medicine is consistently maintained by a particular axiomatic premise: persistent desire for total control over birth, life and death (Witness the recent expose on medical eugenics in Sweden reported in the LA *Times* (1999). Swedish physicians, between 1930–1974, systemically and routinely sterilized thousands of innocent people deemed mentally ill). Axiology speaks to the notion of values (e.g., truth morality). In the United States, both fear and intolerance of population growth among the poor and people of color, as well as a peculiar insecurity about white identity, drives a scientific rationalism to irrational distortions, which take root in particular values and meanings of public health practice.

The problems with public health, as practiced by the modem health care industry, are diverse. The basic cause of the disquiet centers in public health's frustrating inability to make inroads against conditions that disable, kill, and undermine quality of life. When treating conditions of "unknown etiology" and particularly the complex life-process disorders that give rise to chronic problems, illness or disease, much broader systemic issues take primacy. It is fundamental that the social position of African Americans be addressed. Modern public health practice has adopted and reflected the culture of modern medicine (King and Nobles, 1996). Implicit to this culture is a certain ontology (existence as individualism), which defines a certain type of human relationship involving hierarchy, sharp divisions of

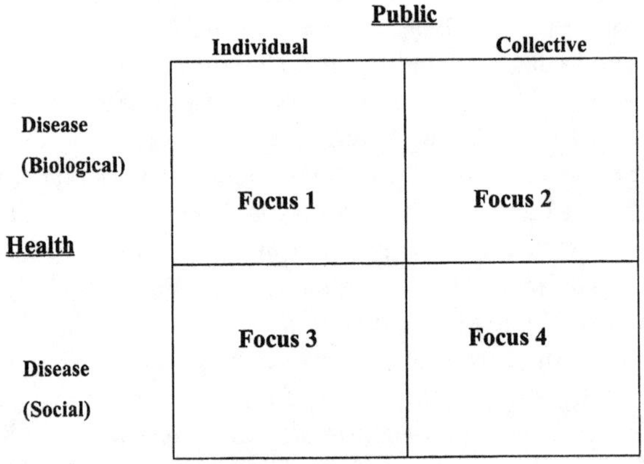

Figure 20.   Conception of the primary focus of public health as represented in the dominant literature.

work, an even narrower specialization. This culture also defines how knowledge is gained (epistemology), and even narrower specialization. This cultural orientation also defines how knowledge (epistemology) is gained and distributed. In this case, the emphasis is on scientific rationalism and the written word. Finally, this cultural direction delineates the values placed on human existence (axiology). In this case, African Americans are marginalized in this world that is divided by those who know and have, and those who do not know and do not have. African Americans and the poor are relegated to the second category (Williams, 1990).

Modern medicine can be clearly characterized as being guided by a specific cultural approach serving those who know and have. These three characteristics, reflected in the relationships inside the public health system, constitute the "culture of public health" in which medicine is made regnant, and fetishized, while humans (at least African Americans) are reified and marginalized as objects. Simply adding new and critically important variables to an existing paradigm without examination of its inviolate assumptions and principles is an exercise in futility. A classic recent example of this is HIV prevention. Models, developed for and by gay white males and serving that population quite effectively, are now being applied to populations of color without their involvement or consent. Now in a "magical effort" to serve African Americans, the church has been pulled in to undertake actions without a legitimate theoretical base from which to address the problem.

It is the central thesis of this paper that health problems confronting the African American population must be paradigmatically reconfigured. This reconfiguration must place the person, and not medicine, as the subject of the health discourse. The basis of this discourse must be authentic culture. This discourse must be thought of in moral, political and social terms, as in biological development terms, within the framework of this authentic culture in the service of all humans.

Core Issue for Alternative Models

The Challenges

Health practitioners of whatever approach, and health care itself, would be better off remembering the prayer of the great physician and philosopher Moses Maimonides eight centuries ago: "Give me the courage to realize my daily mistakes so that tomorrow I shall be able to see and understand in a better light what I could not comprehend in the dim light of yesterday" (Cecil, 1982: xhii).

At the beginning of the 21st century we are still confronted with the "daily mistakes" that generate the persistent problem of the "color line" (DuBois, 1970) that marginalizes a great segment of the citizens of the United States. Health professionals must become courageous in undertaking the challenges to remove the marginalization that is central to the production of excess mortality and morbidity of African Americans. In the fixed "personal hygiene" culture of public health, African Americans are excluded. Consider the men who called Copernicus mad because of his courage to proclaim that the earth moved. For them, this was not possible because what they meant by "earth" was their fixed position (Kuhn, 1970). The cultural hegemony of a public health model that "fixes" the African American into a marginalized status is equally as problematic. So, despite accumulating failures under the assault of evidence of public health approaches, what has collapsed is not the approaches, but the people the approaches are presumed to serve. How many millions of malaria cases would have been avoided if Sir Richard Burton had not dismissed as a "naive view" the indigenous Somali representation that mosquitoes caused malaria?

In the European "fixed position," the cause was "miasmas." How many millions in urban populations could enjoy an improvement in the quality of their lives if, for example, funding was not so skewed in the direction of the search for genetic markers? In the European fixed position mindset, the subject is medicine and the cause is genetic. The seduction of gene mapping has a host of new medical treatment crusaders searching for genetic markers for everything, from abuse to Zen. Meanwhile, public health development, driven by medicine, plays a waiting game for the genetic maps to be completed.

Perhaps the greatest manifestation of the "fixed position" can be observed at NIH review committee meetings and in the research citations of researchers who build a career on the backs of the poor community. In most instances, the authentic work of African American researchers is completely ignored. In the interim, the equivalent of small nuclear bombs explode yearly in communities throughout the United States without a single word, while America waits (Navarro, 1984). There cannot be much doubt that modem medicine's paradigms and the resulting methodology are failing in public health on the most critical front: the spread of chronic disabling problems, illnesses and killer diseases. What Copernicus established was a whole new way regarding the relationship of the earth to the sun, one that changed the meaning of both the earth and motion. How does one place African American at the center of their health universe? The crisis of health in the African American community is too grave to ignore. Once again, the spotlight is on African American scholars, even as we are called "deluded," to declare a challenge to flawed Eurocentric paradigms. Our task is not to "paint the white doll black" (King, 1998) or even negate the European mindset. The real challenge is to make the quantum leap over the persistent negation of our reality, and to recover the essence of that which is human, in order to articulate models more grounded in the reality of the people to be served. This requires a radical departure from the notion of health as individual hygiene understood in terms of scientific rationalism.

Engagement in the serious task of negating African American marginalization is a highly political process. The notions of eugenics and European hegemony must be absolutely rejected. African Americans must become subject participants in the process in all events that affect their lives. The recent World Health Organization's definition of health promotion recognizes the need for such a political process to address a new direction in the approach to public health. Its approach states that:

> Health promotion is the process of enabling individuals and communities to increase control over the determinants of health and thereby improve their health. Such a process requires the direct involvement of individuals and communities in the achievement of change combined with political action directed towards the creation of an environment conducive to health. (WHO, 1994)

A sketch of a conceptually different approach to viewing Public Health, in contrast to the approach in Figure 20, is presented in Figure 21.

Figure 21 represents an alternative view of public health. In this view "public consists of people-I relationship"—individuals embedded in family, family rooted in community, community based in society. Health is viewed as quality of relationships that affect biological, psychological, social and spiritual well-being. The validity of epistemological claims depends on this understanding that health's essential quality is in relationships. Health is represented in unity as one line, polarized to indicate negative ($-$) or optimum ($+$) health relationships.

However, both of these together do not complete the picture of public health. What is required is the "ground," or context, on which they stand. Context permits the authentic relationship of the public with its heath existence—political, cultural, ecological, and economic.

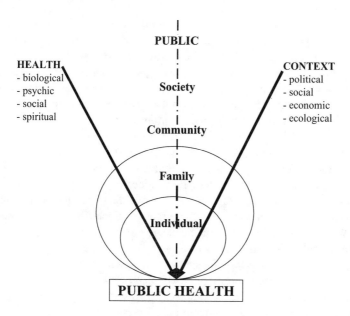

Figure 21. An alternative view of public health as the health of relationships.

This is represented by a single line, again polarized into negative and positive, not as objective sum and substance but as perceptions of the "public" of the context.

The Implications for Alternative Approaches

The point of departure for Figure 21 is the "public" at the center of the discourse on public health. This has implications for developing alternative approaches to public health. The most fundamental issue for any new approach, consistent with the WHO, 1994 declaration, must be the inclusion and control by African Americans over the determinant of heir health. We must locate a whole new way regarding the relationship of the African American to health. Social status, culture and behavior are all critical variables in this new culture of public health. The health status of African Americans is influenced not only by the unique pattern of exposure to stressors based on the African Americans' social status in the U.S. but also by the way African Americans, given their historical values and meanings (culture), behave in response to stress and life's adversities in rapidly changing society. Three issues become critical for new approaches: the primacy of culture, the reality of relationships, and the nexus of behavior change.

The Primacy of Culture

Culture is the first leg of the "public health stool" (Gergen et al., 1997; Nobles and King, 2000). Yet culture is often dismissed in urban public health. There are three dimensions to the culture proposition. One dimension attends to the group as "public". Another dimension focuses on health as a medium of exchange. The third dimension spotlights the environment as context—political, ecological, economic and spiritual.

In the first instance, the public refers to African Americans. African Americans are not only treated as social pariahs, but also as having no legitimate culture. This is the core of African American negation. Implicit in mainstream thinking about the words "African Americans" are a series of relations—color, class position, roles in society, etc.—in relation to something else: the dominant white community. It is the comparison, in the South African sense, in which the highest position for African Americans is that of honorary whites. This is a root problem. African Americans, in anthropological, social, and political contexts, constitute a culture. Over time, African Americans have developed a set of values, beliefs, meanings and practices—and, by extension, a way of health. If one is to create authentic public health for African Americans, the primacy of culture must be affirmed.

The second dimension focuses in the culture of public health, itself, as health. In establishing a new public health practice, the issue of the individual driven by a genetic epistemology that characterizes dominant models must be confronted. What has dominated the literature in the medial model paradigm has been the individual "at-risk". Current medical practice emphasizes factors that, at best, identify biological intrapersonal factors (weak organs systems), or psychological intrapersonal factors (belief, cognitions, attitude, intentions, skills) as determinants of health outcomes. Such descriptive data attend to the individual. The data, therefore, encourage and suggest that any intervention program aiming to improve health outcomes needs to change the individual by targeting his/her personal characteristics and behaviors (Rogers et al., 1993). For example most providers of health care services to urban minority populations report that patients not only have multiple illness diagnosis, but also some "comorbid" reality including homelessness, substance abuse, migrant status, or illiteracy (Fulmer et al., 1992), as well as unemployment and low income (Amick, 1994; Terris, 1983). Yet the intervention remains focused exclusively on issues of emotional disturbance, cognitive impairment, motivation and depression.

The third dimension of culture is context, the web of relationships between the public and social reality. The present health conditions of African Americans are not acts of nature, but are defined through historically and socially specific human interaction in society. There is a series of interactive exchanges between African Americans and the social environment. One of these concerns health. The African American historical experience in health begins in Africa. This experience is extended to the U.S. where the relationship between African Americans, the health establishment, and the community and social environment is not an isolated individual phenomena, as scientific rationalism would have one believe, but the product of a history of relationships. Culture is the mediating construct in the web of relationships (Nobles and King, 2000). The health of all people must be examined from the vantage point of this web of relationships. Negating this web by negating culture is at the core of the production of incoherence and therefore illness. The challenge is to offer an alternative to resolve the person's incoherence in the world, addressing the perpetual crisis of loss of voice and authentic identity (King and Nobles, 1997). Culture is the mediating force that maintains unity and coherence of the web of relationships. The subject of culture must be placed at the center of the discourse on health in addressing an alternative model. In the clash between the Public Health culture dominated by "psychological genetics" and African Americans, if the African American person's health circumstance is to be adequately understood and addressed, then it must be done from the vantage point of culture. If the assumption continues that the African American is without culture, then there is not even a possibility of resolving issues at the level of culture mediation. In the absence of the mediation of culture, there is no coherence and therefore, no health.

The Reality of Relationship

How one conceptualizes relationships has direct implications for the issue of "risk". Where one places risk has implications for development of an alternative public health approach.

In the first public health models—the quarantine model of hygiene—risk was seen in terms of space. Lines were drawn between healthy and unhealthy spaces such as houses, town, or ships. The second public health model shifted to concerns with sanitation. This model identified risks to health in terms of the space between the body and non-corporal, eternal space. The third public health model shifted to personal hygiene, one that developed along with the rise of the medical model, the focus is placed on personal cleanliness and behavior such as exercise, eating *and* smoking. Within this framework risks to health are located *within* individual space (Ogden, 1995).

In addressing the limitations of the psychological genetic paradigm dominated by individualism, researchers have begun to emphasize a fourth model of public health that emphasizes health promotion, lifestyle, and ecological dangers. Within this framework, risks to health exist in the spaces within and between individuals as well as between individuals and the socially engineered environment (Ogden, 1995). Researchers have begun to emphasize the consequences of organizational and community support, the role of the church, and the importance of employment opportunity in the complex relationship between the individual and his/her social, physical and cultural environments. This viewpoint, stressing socially situated human environment transactions has been called the "ecological perspective" (Bronfonbrenner, 1979) or "web of causation". It shifts the focus from individual responsibility for maintaining health to the economic, political and structural elements in society that encourage, produce and support unhealthy environmental conditions (Stein, 1992). Implicit in the ecological perspective is a refocus of attention, away from individual and individual choices (intra-individual factors) that affect behavior, and toward environmental determinants of behavior (Clitheroe et al., 1998).

Despite what appears as a radical departure from "personal hygiene" notions of public health, approaches have not kept up with this new "web of interaction" notion of risk being interconnected with living community. Public health seems unable to shake free of this notion of risk "within" the individual even as it struggles to include the larger environment. Although this idea of "the web of interaction" is suggested as a framework in public health practice, the individual has simply been reconfigured through surveillance that again emphasizes and places the burden on personal control over lifestyle. In the reconfiguring, what has emerged is a new "individual psychological genetics" under the label of "health behavior change."

The Nexus of Behavior Change

Health behavior change has become a dominant theme in public health approaches. Great emphasis is placed on lifestyle changes. Illness prevention studies have relied heavily on models of behavior influence, and in particular, communications tailored to facilitate movement through the stages of change. The message is this: The car is speeding; there is no stop sign; learn the lifestyle (behavior change) of safe street crossing. Below are some of the models widely used to address chronic health problems (smoking, cancer, HIV/AIDS, hypertension, substance abuse, and violence, etc):

The Transtheoretical or "Stages of Change" Model (Prochaska and DiClemente, 1983), which focuses on cognitive behavior. According to cognitive behavioral theory, change progresses as the individual moves from the pre-contemplation stage (not even thinking about changing a specific behavior), to the contemplation stage (starting to consider, but not yet actually acting on a behavior change course), followed by a preparation stage (preparing to change the behavior in the near future), then to the action stage (making the initial steps toward behavior change), and finally, to the maintenance stage (maintaining behavior change and not even thinking about reverting).

The Health Belief Model (Becker, 1974) proposes that individuals are most likely to take preventive action when they perceive themselves to be susceptible to some adverse outcome. They believe that outcome would be severe for them, and see more reasons to make the change than impediments to making the change.

The Theory of Protection Motivation (Maddox and Rogers, 1983) likewise recognizes the importance of personal vulnerability and disease severity. It also stresses the importance of the individual's perception of the effectiveness of available risk reduction options (similar to perceived benefits in the health belief model), as well as his or her sense of personal power to initiate and implement risk reduction activities (related to the health belief model's perceived barriers).

Social Learning Theory (Bandura, 1977) proposes that when people believe they are able to take some action and believe that action will lead to desirable outcomes, they are more likely to do so.

The Theory of Reasoned Action (Fishbein and Aizen, 1985) describes the process and conditions under which health or other behaviors are acquired and modified, focusing on the importance of an individual's attitude toward performing an action, (such as using condoms) as well as the individual's perceptions of how a significant other feels about his or her performing that action.

These preventive intervention approaches are narrowly focused on individual behavior change. Despite this narrow focus, they should not be negated. In fact, the models are excellent exemplars of a culturally consistent "Eurocentric" public health approach. Unfortunately, although they make no claims to universality, they are applied as if they were. These models rely quite heavily on cognition or efficacy. These are decontextualized variables, and in the absence of the relationship to cultural context, severely limiting. Such approaches, despite reported short-term successful outcomes (e.g., Rogers et al., 1993; Stanton, 1997) must necessarily be non-transformative as they fail to go beyond mere descriptions of health consciousness. If used without modification, the unintended consequences of the models would be to further advance the marginalization of the "other" cultures, African Americans in particular.

The line of approach, investigating predictors of behavior change among urban minorities, dominated by personal influence paradigms, has necessarily not produced desired public health results for African Americans (Altpeter et al., 1998). Attributing behavior change problems exclusively to the individual not only has biased providers against the poor and urban multi-cultural populations, but also unwittingly has limited providers' willingness to make needed changes in health care services (Weinstein et al., 1998). Deeply ingrained in each formulation is the focus on the individual (cognition, perceptions, personal vulnerability belief, and attitude).

The very idea of the autonomous individual is very seductive. One cannot really fault the theory of personal responsibility and personal life style. It is somewhat of a "mother and apple pie" tradition. Yet it must be fully recognized as producing an epistemological problem. Such theoretical approaches detach illness and health from historically specific struggles in which they are embedded. This dismisses society (history, experiences, relationships to the social order) as a fundamental contributing element in the discussion of disease, and fosters an incomplete analysis of the problem, resulting in incomplete data for addressing the health problems of African Americans. The complete data set to address the health condition of African Americans has yet to be developed. The concept of relationships and culture has been superseded by artifact, to the negation of the substance of African American culture. If we are to advance from narrow individualism-driven paradigms, we must engage an approach grounded in culture. If the African American person is to recover health, then the person must regain coherence. If s/he is to return to coherence, s/he must reclaim culture.

A Framework for Authentic Models

From all the other "races" of humanity (the Egyptians, Indians, Greeks, Romans, Teutons) the "African American" writes DuBois,

> is a sort of seventh son, born with a veil, and gifted with second-sight in this American world, a world which yields him no true self-consciousness, but only lets him see himself through the revelation of the other world. It is a peculiar sensation, this double-consciousness and this sense of always looking at oneself through the eyes of others (DuBois, 1970).

DuBois was correct. The ruptured nature of the cultural context of the African American person has implications for excess deaths. In constructing an alternative there is an absolute necessity to define methods to identify, reflect, and address the African American person's dominant opposing internal motivational currents (Stem, 1992) or "contradiction of double aims" (DuBois, 1970) produced by disrupted cultural continuity and persistent social negation. In a monograph commissioned by the Centers for Disease Control, King and Nobles (1996) argued for an approach in which a culturally constructed self in a web of relationships replaces individualism. They articulated the following position:

> Models are formulated and created within and in relation to particular cultural relationships that are a product of historical movement. A model is a theoretical construction through which cultural categories (ontology, axiology and epistemology) and concepts are articulated as abstract principles in an attempt to specify and comprehend the concrete principles that are the governing process of any historical movement. The historical movement of a process is located within and by means of the material and nonmaterial relations between an object, which is in a dynamic state of movement, and a subject, which continually and constantly formulates a cultural praxis towards effectively transforming its relations with the object. Hence, a theoretical model, if it is concretely and historically conscious of its process of creation and movement, is a corrective instrument that attempts to apprehend the reciprocity between an object and a subject. The reciprocity between a subject and an object is a product of and within historical relations (p. 25).

Inherent in this declaration are the principles that form the basis of an alternative approach to public health. Central and fundamental to this are the roles of culture (Gergen et al., 1997; Nobles and King, 1997) as the organizing framework upon which all actions rest. King and Nobles (1997) coined the concept of "culturecology" to capture this cultural framing.

Parameters of the Culturecology Framing

The following is a summary of the central assumption, basic tenants, and methods of an authentic culturecology model. The details are published elsewhere (King and Nobles, 1996, 1997).

Basic Assumption
There are four primary assumptions:

1. Public Health is a cultural phenomenon. The basis of all phenomena is relationship—a person nested in a triadic set of relationships (web-of-relationships) consisting of the person, his/her community and his/her environment (Haslam, 1994). The sum of relationships (unit or web or relationships) of any phenomenon is called culture; culture is the defining substance of all human action (e.g., Carruthers, 1995; Hilliard, 1976). Public Health is no exception. Public Health is a transactionally produced condition in any unit of relationships. What defines and maintains the unit as a unit in this web of relationships is culture. Culture is a functional, internally consistent system of beliefs, attitudes, values, expectations and norms/patterns of conduct. What maintains the unity is the relationship within and between the person and the community/environment. In the person dimension (which is never independent of context), culture directs his/her level of autonomous capacity for self-organization as well as that of self-restoration. In the community dimension (which is never independent of persons), culture directs the level of social and economic support and the balance in relation to ecology and faith. Coherence, and therefore health, depends on the availability, use and balance of health-protective and health restoring factors in the web of relationships. The first inviolate assumptions that the individual's health is a relational event that can be best understood as a situationally bound unit of relationships (organic, psychological, family, social, political and spiritual) in which culture is the unifying link [cultural faming]. A culturally framed event, then, is one that is defined in terms of its own reality, system of values and ways of knowing (King and Davis, 1999).

2. Bonds as the basis of the unity as represented by Culture. This is the second assumption. Bonds are the dimensions internal to culture. A bond is a historical-cognitive emotional structure (connection) that has clear functions in everyday functioning of a unit of relationships. The web of relationships reflects bonds to personal, conventional, social, and spiritual order. If culture represents the structure of a system in unity, then bonds represent or are forms of "glue" that maintain the ties or attachments, and therefore the function or dysfunction of the web of relationships. Cultural framing prompts the articulation of the organic set of bonds as the defining reality at any given moment for any given relation. Using a positive stretch of imagination, one might conceptualize, as physical medicine has, that the individual in relation to him/herself is the smallest event unit, consisting of a set of relationships held together by bonds. This conception can never be the case in Public Health. The smallest event unit in Public health is the individual in context (see Figure 21), held in the relationship by bonds (King and Fluker, 1999).

3. The third assumption is that there are four primary bonds (Fiske, 1993). These bonds are fundamental and universal, and assume different forms as a function of development of the relational unit. Development of the unit can be influenced internally (e.g., a local campaign to provide well-baby care to pregnant drug-abusing mothers) or externally (e.g., the removal of Federal funds for health care to pregnant, unwed mothers). These bonds can be conceptualized as follows:

- *Affinity bonds*. The need for collective belonging, or solidarity, and intimacy based on memory. These bonds grow from the memory of childhood (feeding, comfort, protection) and are based on the need for security and trust.
- *Obligation bonds*. The drive to establish rules according to status markers such as deeds (good or bad), age, skill, knowledge, class, social position, race. These bonds

are based on the meaning of power, order and control, and grow from the spirit nature of relationships and the need for accountability, duty, responsibility, and moral commitment.

- *Assurance bonds.* Bonds based on the organization on common sets of values of exchange, such as vocation, production, money, goods, materials, or intellectual work. The emphasis is on good return on investment or time. Social transaction is based on costs and benefits. Assurance bonds are based on the search or need for competence, mastery, or autonomy.
- *Harmony bonds.* These are the bonds governed by the search for fairness and rhythm. They are the ties organizing the construction and interpretation of relationships in strictly impartial terms. As an example of this is the search for equity. (Nobles and King, 1997). These focus on reciprocity, fairness as primary values. Such bonds are based on the motivation for justice, fairness and balance.

Every relationship can be defined by these bonds. Bonds are either present or absent. When they are present, they are either strong or weak, health enhancing or health-compromising. Bonds characterize the nature of the event. If we assume that all people require relationships that respect them, produce good self-esteem, promote knowledge or worth, and respect from others, and good feelings about where they are gong and of their chances of getting there, then the question becomes: What bonds inform what we observe as health outcomes from given webs of relationships?

4. The fourth and final assumption is that the essence of an event/phenomenon is not in the phenomenon itself, but in its web of relationships. This implies that the unit of analysis in the examination of any public health occurrence must be the web of health relationships in that event. Fundamental to understanding the event as a relationship is the nature of the bonds in culturally framed web. Bonds constitute the essence. It is within the framework the person's (family's, community's) bond to a larger reality that factors (psychological, social, ecological, spiritual) central in setting the stage for modifying bonds and therefore the conditions for behavior change—occur. For the person, family, or community, this may include perceptions of being at risk in a given relationship, perceived benefits of a change in that relationship or the confidence that the necessary change in their relationship can be made (self-efficacy). Also significant is the symbolic and real role that the relationship plays in a person's life (King and Nobles, 1996) in the context of a given historical reality. It is from this culturally framed web of relationships that one can better understand the bonds that promote autonomous motivation (Deci and Ray, 1985) for behavior change in the individual, family, community or society.

Principles

- The presence of strong health-enhancing bonds in all four bonding domains is necessary to optimum health and the prevention of illness. For the person, the stronger health-enhancing the bonds, the stronger the formation of a collective self-identity as a part of community. Therefore, it is less likely that the person will engage in relationships that involve risk factors for a host of negative health outcomes.
- The same statement is true and can be applied to the family and the community/society.
- Conversely, the presence of health-compromising bonds, or the absence or weakness of autonomous bonds (to personal, spiritual and the conventional social order), predict a greater likelihood of the person engaging in risk factors for a host of

negative health outcomes for him/herself, community or society. King and Nobles argue that African American health relations are significantly compromised by a society that has historically negated [Maafa] (Ani, 1994) African American bonds to society (conventional social order). What allows the African American to survive is the positive [Maafa] (Ani, 1994) remnants of historical bonds to cultural history (spiritual connections). These remnant subsets of Ma'at are necessary for survival, but not sufficient for mastery and optimal health. The development of mastery depends on strong heath-enhancing bonds to both self and society.

Methodology. In this exploration of an initial summary sketch of methodology for a culturecological modeling in a public health approach, the focus is primarily on subject, design, and general procedural steps.

Subject of Analysis. The methodology of the culturecological model focuses on the web of relationships as the unit of analysis and the subject for exploration. The unit is always the nested person, situated in material space, situated in nonmaterial space in a web of relationships. The unifying link is culture. Let us examine, for example, the health issue of diabetes. The subject of analysis is the set of bonds that maintains the particular relationship to the production of diabetes—Diabetes is an outcome of his set of bonds. Diabetes never becomes the active subject; it remains an "object." Examination of the relational bonds of the web of relationships producing diabetes leads to questions about the bonds of a whole person in whole relationships, the roles in the unit (not in the person) of various bonds. We are then in a position to observe the many outcomes of the "bonding" of which one outcome is diabetes.

Design. The model suggests that the first step of design of intervention always begins with careful work in identifying or locating the smallest web of relationship or cultural event of the whole person in whole contexts, such as in the case of AIDS. In developing a design, the question to be asked is for a target group (e.g., youth 15–25 years) is a web of relationships question. In what social situation (school, street, dropouts, poverty, etc.)? In what nonmaterial space (resistance to authority, fun seeking, woman/manhood expression, oppression) constitutes our unit of analysis? Then we pose the question: what consistent pattern of bonds maintains both positive and negative outcomes for the unit? Of these bonds, which are health enhancing, and which are illnesses producing?

The second step is cultural framing, which requires both cultural sensitivity and competence. The frame consists of the representation of the types, strength and valence of bonds present in the web of relationships. The central methodology for the discovery of bonds within cultural framing is the use of narrative (King and Fluker, 1998).

The third step is the participation of the subject in change, recognizing that what is to be changed are the nature of bonds within the web-of-relations, which maintain outcomes that are health compromising.

In a chapter such as this, only a sketch of the methodology is possible. A more extensive discussion on this methodology is presented in King and Nobles (1996).

Procedural Steps: Here is a guide framework for the most basic notions of approach:

1. The first task is always to undertake, from a culturecology frame of reference, critical study of the nature and epidemiology of the basic units of relationships that produce high-risk behaviors and the converse, of relationships that preserve health and well-being. The analysis must involve both if one is to work from the historical strengths of the

public to be served. This critical search for the basic relationship must be consistent with see-ing the relationship in the context (political, ecological, economic, social) of the larger web of relationships. In addressing the pubic health issue of adolescent health, for example, too often attention is paid to outcomes such as HIV/AIDS, or smoking. The outcome (some form of compromised health, e.g. lung cancer) is not the subject, it is object. The subject is the rela-tionship set (youth in relation to tobacco, authority, industry, etc.) that produces this object outcome. The task of critical analysis is to define this set as comprehensively as possible.

2. The second intervention task begins with selecting and specifying the set of rela-tionships, the relationship of primary focus (as subject) that produces the behavior leading to the outcome (as object). Careful research must be undertaken to identify and define this basic unit of study, intervention, or discourse. This is really a political decision based in cost-benefit analysis both economic and scientific. Having specified the key relationship of interest, the task then becomes the thorough exploration in this dominant attributable relationship, the bonds that maintain both the health indicators and the relative risk indi-cators. In addressing the public health issue of adolescent smoking, for example, the ques-tion must be raised about what bonds maintain the relationship of primary concern (e.g., relationship to cigarettes or relationship to peers).

3. The third task is one of strategic goal setting. The public health approach always must seek to formulate goals and strategic direction for intervention in conjunction with the other relationship (national and community policies, and priorities for prevention and health promotion) in which the primary relations are embedded. In other words, the primary relationship of intervention may be youth in relation to cigarettes. This unit must be embedded in the community, e.g., its economics, and resources and the society includ-ing its policies toward tobacco industry. The strategic direction should guide the develop-ment of goals for health promotion, health protection, prevention services, or clinical intervention.

4. The fourth task is to develop a culturecological intervention program appropriate to and in conjunction with, the subject population. That development, as a result of the analysis in #2 above, the cultural framing that should guide the intervention to include tim-ing (primary, secondary, tertiary prevention; level personal relations, family relations, community relations, etc.), and desired outcomes. The desired outcome usually falls into one of three categories: changing the existing relational complex, establishing a new relational context, or both.

5. Finally, it is necessary to situate the entire enterprise in a research-based context to inform all relationships within and between units, and put in place intervention, imple-mentation and evaluation protocols to include:

a. Process research
b. Pilot research
c. Efficacy trial
d. Effectiveness trial
e. Data analysis and dissemination

Case Study Using the Approach

In this final section of a culture critique of Public Health we suggest, by way of a brief case study overview, how the application of a culturecology framework redefines the idea of public health. The details of this case study are presented elsewhere (Hinkle, 1997).

An opportunity to use a culturecology allocation of $2,000,000 to improve the health status of California's low-income African-American, Latino, Asian and American Indian youth 10 to 14 years old.

The author of this paper, as chairperson of an eight-member trustee board mandated by the court, set out with the board to design a plan to improve the health status among poor ethnic minority youth. Here is an outline of a culturecological framework process we undertook in a very successful effort to bring about changes in the health determinants of over 10,000 youth in the state of California. Recently, the Centers for Disease Control and Prevention and USDA, in a joint effort adopted the approach developed from this work for a national pilot study designed to address childhood obesity in African Americans.

Here is a summary of the group's public health approach to the health of poor children age 10–14 years.

The General Problem

First we explored the general problem of the health of children and its significance as a public health issue.

Over the last two decades, it has been consistently demonstrated that alcohol, poor nutrition and fitness, and smoking contribute to over 70% of the mortality and morbidity among African Americans. The health status behaviors of adults have their origins in childhood. Children and adolescents who repeatedly present with complaints have become burdens/encumbrances to health care professionals, as they significantly overuse primary health care resources. Their subjective symptoms may be the best predictor of subsequent morbidity and mortality, and hence cannot continue to be ignored.

What are the sources of these early symptoms as represented by youth problem behavior and unhealthy life styles (Clitheroe, 1998)?

What is learned during the developmental years is integral to the development of a foundation on which adult health behaviors will be formed. Yet little attention is paid to the child-environment relations that over time inform the health behavior (nutritional intake, fitness, smoking and drug use, as examples) that promote or compromise health. How does one engage the child's relational context to permit the development of alternative bonds to behaviors and practices that are health-promoting and disease-preventing? An understanding of the relational bonds that inform the process of optimum health requires recognition of factors that contribute to and maintain bonds (patterns of interactions) in human health development.

The Primary Relationship of Focus. The first step of the intervention is undertaking a critical, culturally framed analysis. Evidence seems to support the existence of organized patterns of adolescent risk behaviors (Jessor et al., 1991, 1998). The culturecology model directs us to examine, within a cultural frame, the relationships that produce the behaviors. Consistent with culture-context perspective, adolescents can be characterized as a sub-cultural group within the culture. It is a perspective that suggests a more comprehensive concern with the entire array of adolescent risk relationships, and simultaneously promotes efforts to understand and alter the circumstances that produce and sustain risk relationships in adolescence. These relationships (structures of behaviors), taken together, reflect an adolescent's way of being-and-relating in the world. The relationships suggest a social ecology of adolescent life as a distinct sub-culture, an ecology that provides normative expectations, beliefs, and values. The different risk relationships can serve the same functions. For example, both illicit drug use and precocious sexual activity can provide a way of affirming independence from parents. Depending on the research, interest and resources, the public health professional selects a primary relationship as the subject of focus. In our case, we chose to focus on the relations' attendant to nutrition and fitness, or physical activity, as the primary unit of analysis in considering health status.

From the analysis, this is what followed:

1. *Subject*: We accessed the units of intervention with a focused strategy on low income youth communities using the following parameters: age, family income, culture, health problems of youth, food distribution, opportunity for physical activity, daily activities around food, and reported adolescent problems. The identification yielded over 1,000 communities, both rural and urban. Schools were not directly targeted. From this population, we selected 160 of these youth clusters for follow-up action. The action primarily consisted of identification of key informant and responsible adult leaders, face to face information-sharing meeting at regional meeting across the state, and information mailer/responses to information requests. This action effort was specifically focused on establishing a relationship and building trust among a network of influential leaders and community-based organizations to engage in planning a health promotion strategy. This was accomplished through problem definition and strategic direction, approach to problem resolution, attainment of vision and resource allocation. The issues of nutrition and physical fitness were not on the agenda of over 90% of the groups identified. Therefore, we targeted this as a fundamental discourse at the inception the physical fitness were not on the agenda of over 90% of the groups identified. Therefore, we targeted this as a fundamental discourse at the inception, meaning and value of health and wellness. These are the critical values of the group. What are the expectations for adolescents?

The fundamental discourse began to emerge around the relationship of focus: the adolescent relationship to nutrition and fitness. This was immediately followed up, using a focus group method and in-depth exploration of the adolescent-nutrition/fitness relationship and its connection to health; local realities (available food supply and food services), cultural realities ethnic foods and expectations); national standards (e.g., USDA's "5 a-day" recommendation).

2. Each of the 160 groups then was invited to submit an application request to initiate action on improving the health status of poor adolescents, focused on the issue of nutrition and fitness. The groups could request planning or program implementation funding. The planning funds ($10,000) were designed to help structure a culturecological plan for the defined target community. The implementation funds were designed to support implementation of community groups that already had what closely resembled a culturecological plan in place. Planning awards were for nine (9) months. We anticipated further funding for up to 50% of the planning grantees for 1–3 year implementation efforts. The implementation awards ($50–75,000 annually) were intended to support strategies for recreating or establishing positive bond around nutrition and fitness. The guidelines for program development and criteria for funding closely followed the protocol questions raised by the culturecological model. In developing their approaches, grantees were required:

- To demonstrate use of culturecological-specific interventions (cultural framing) to overcome historical impediments and to advance youth sustainability;
- To evaluate the feasibility of the Intervention;
- To institutionalize and create the possibility of transferability of program elements to similar groups in the state

Results: The first three-year effort involved 22 communities that were funded by this effort. The breakdown by groups was as follows:

	African A	Asian	Latino	Am Indian	Mixed
Urban	4	3	3	0	4
Rural	0	I	3	2	2

Youth self-determination was observed as a powerful force across all programs over the life of the project, over 10,000 adolescents participated and were fully empowered in specific youth-generated activities to change the nature of the bond that informed their nutrition and fitness relationships. There were dramatic changes in illness-producing nutrition and physical activity bonds across all groups. Among the more creative examples of activities in changing relationships were:

- Middle school students in rural Monterey County actively engaged their school in deciding how nutrition and physical activity was to be incorporated into their new school-based community enter;
- Youth in Kalasugan County worked with their Community Services Department to create more ethnically appropriate nutrition and physical education class options.
- In Chula Vista, youths are now learning Filipino stick dances as a fitness activity.
- In Santa Paula, a quebradita dance and nutrition class is now taught three times a week. Such new bonds form the basis for new relationship to nutrition.
- American Indian adolescents on the Pauma Reservation in rural San Diego County are learning from tribal elders' traditional Indian games. The youth-sponsored activity at community powwow ceremonies where games are played now includes fresh fruit, vegetables and water as alternatives to the omnipresent fry-bread snack.
- Latino youth in the Colton Soccer League created a peer-driven club that works with local health departments and food stores to provide fruit and vegetables as after-soccer game snacks.
- In San Leandro, Girls Inc. developed a 10-week Afro-centric curriculum built around hip-hop dance that focuses on self-esteem, body image, healthy eating, cooking, and physical activity.

Each group of adolescents was able to engage in a new relationship in the context of nutrition and fitness. Each was able to build capacity, to develop its own self-help materials, worksite strategies, curricula and other nutrition and fitness resources. We have since put these materials together as an adolescent nutrition and fitness resource manual.

Overall we were able to institutionalize an adolescent nutrition and fitness organization (CANFit) in the State of California. CANFit now serves as a grant-giving agency focused on the nutrition and physical fitness of poor youth in California. CDC and USDA, in a new national pilot study focused on adolescent obesity problems have adopted the program model.

Conclusions

The focus of the chapter has been a cultural critique of public health as practiced in urban America. The critique has centered on three primary issues: The nature of the present reality of public health with its emphasis on individuals (public health's ontology); the deification of scientific rationalism as the only method of value (public health's axiology) in understanding the public's health; the emphasis on knowledge gained from events internal to the individual (public health's epistemology) rather than knowledge gained from the study of relationships. We suggested an alternative based on recasting the subject (and thus the discourse) of public health as the *culturally framed relationship*, one that seeks an understanding of the event in terms of its own reality, system of values, and ways of knowing (King and Davis, 1999).

This chapter began by addressing the devastating state of health and quality of life for African Americans. The medical model of public health would have us believe that the lifestyle of African Americans is the primary contributing factor to their disease condition. A culturecology position emphasizes the reality of the history of relations of African Americans in the U.S.A culturecology approach examines the values placed on the lives of African Americans, who are yet to be paid for their labor as slaves and have now become expendable, and subjected to new forms of slavery. A culturecology overture helps to uncover the strengths and knowledge of a people who have suffered centuries of abuse and still survive. We may discover that, far from being random or idiosyncratic, the knowledge, attitudes, and lifestyles of the African American can be viewed as consistent and understandable responses to problems associated with their position in the social structure and life chances.

The culturecology framework does not seek to romanticize the African reality. It is a constant reminder, as Brother Wade Nobles reminds us, that we are "cultural substance." As such, the framework demands a continuous critique, exposing the bankruptcy and the lack of integrity of models or paradigms of human or social transformation (public health included) that places culture as an additive variable. It is cultural understanding itself that may inform what appears to be the resistance to the influence of modem day constructs of public health. Such a resistance from the vantage point of cultural understanding, in such a context as ours, may in fact a sign of health, an effort to protect secure relationships (even though illness-producing). These are people who may sense a future no different from their present or their past, and who feel their existence and hence their survival, is threatened by interventions that lead them to adopt the reality, values and knowledge of completely irrelevant, nonfunctional codes seeped in Eurocentric culture. It was not too long ago that Frantz Fanon warned us, in his book *The Wretched of the Earth* (1963. Dag-254),

> Humanity is waiting for something other from us than such an imitation, which would be almost an obscene caricature. For Europe, for ourselves and for humanity, [young scholars], we must turn over a new leaf, we must work out new concepts, and try to set afoot a new man.

References

Altpeter, M., Earp, J.A., and Schopler, J.H. (1998). Promoting breast cancer screening in rural, African American communities: The "science and art" of community health promotion. *Health and Social Work*, 23(2): pp. 104–105.

Amick, R. et al. (Eds.) (1994) *Why Are Some People Healthy and Others Not?* New York: Adeline DeGruyter.

Ani, M. (1994) *Yurugu*: An African-centered critique of European cultural thought and behavior. NY: African World Press.

Bandura, A. (1977). Self-efficacy: Toward a unifying theory of behavior change. *Psychological Review*, 84: pp. 191–215.

Beatty and John. (1995). Cultural perceptions of life and death. *Spirit versus Scalpel: Traditional Healing and Modern Psychotherapy*. (Leonore Loeb Adler, B. Runi Mukherji, Eds.) Westport, CT: Bergin & Garvey/ Greenwood Publishing, pp. 13–24.

Becker, M.H. (ed). (1974). *The health belief model and personal behavior*. Thorofare, NJ: Charles B. Slack.

Beeker, C., Guenther-Grey, C., and Raj, A.A. (1998). Community Empowerment Paradigm Drift and The Primary Prevention of HIV/AIDS. *Social Science and Medicine*, 46(7): pp. 831–42.

Blazer, D. (1982). Social support and mortality in an elderly community population. *American Journal of Epidemiology*. 115: pp. 684–694.

Bronfonbrenner, V. (1979). *The Ecology of Development*, Massachusetts: Harvard University Press.

Brownell, Kelly D. Cohen, and Lisa R. (1995) Adherence to dietary regimens: components of effective interventions. *Behavioral Medicine*, 20 (n4): pp. 155–164.

Carruthers, Jacob. (1995). *MDW NTR Divine Speech*: A Historical Reflection of African Deep Thought From the Time of the Pharaohs to the Present Red Press.

Cassel, J. (1976). The contribution of the social environment to host resistance. *American Journal of Epidemiology*. 104: pp. 107–123.

Centers for Disease Control (1995). *Guidelines for Education and Risk Reduction*, DHSS, Atlanta.

Clitheroe, H.C. Jr., Stokols, Daniel, Zmuidzinas, and Mary. (1998) Conceptualizing the context of environment and behavior. *Journal of Environmental Psychology*, 18 (nl): pp. 103–112.

Deci, E.L. and Ryan, R.M. (1985). *Intrinsic Motivation and self-determination in human behavior*. New York: Plenum.

DuBois, W.E. (1970). *The World and Africa*. New York, NY: Kraus-Thompson Org.

Fanon, F. (1967). *Black Skin, White Masks*. New York: Grove Press.

Fanon, F. (1963). *The Wretched of the Earth*. New York: Evergreen Press.

Fishbein, M. (1979). A theory of reasoned action: Some applications and implications. In H.E. Howe and M.M. Page (Eds.): *Nebraska Symposium on Motivation*. Lincoln, NE: University of Nebraska Press, pp. 61–116.

Fiske, A.P. (1993). *Structures of Social Life: The Four Elementary-Forms of Relations*. New York, NY: Free Press.

Fulmer, H., et al. (1992). Bridging the gap between medicine, public health, and the community: PATCH and the Carney Hospital Experience. *Journal of Health Education*, 23: pp. 167–170.

Gergen, K.J., Gulerce, A., Lock, A., and Misra, G. Psychological Science in Cultural Context. *American Psychologist*, 51(5): pp. 496–503.

Hailer, J.S. (1971). *Outcasts from evolution*. Chicago: University of Illinois Press.

Hahn, R.A. (1995). *Sickness and Healing: An anthropological perspective*. Yale University Press.

Hancock, T. (1999). Future directions in population health. *Canadian Journal of Public Health*, 90(1): pp. 56–70.

Haslam, N. (1994). Categories of social relationship, *Recognition*, 53, pp. 59–90.

Hilliard, A.G. (1976). *Free your mind: Return to the source*. California: Urban Institute Publication.

Hinkle, A. (1977). Community-based nutrition interventions: Reaching adolescents from low-income communities. *Annuals of the New York Academy of Sciences*, 817.

IOM (Institute of Medicine). (1988). *The Future of Public Health*. Washington, DC: National Academy Press.

Jessor, R., Turbin, Mark, S., Costa, and Frances, M. (1998) Risk and protection in successful outcomes among disadvantaged adolescents. *Applied Developmental Science*, v2 (n4): pp. 194–208.

Jessor, R., Donovan, J.E., and Costa, F. (1991). *Beyond adolescence: Problem behavior and young adult development*. New York: Cambridge University Press.

King, L.M. (1998). *Garlic, vinegar and honey: The cultural perspective in developing evaluating community-based health programs*, Atlanta: Council of National Black Churches Conference.

King, L.M. and Davis, D.T. (1999). *Tailored Communication: A culture framework for HIV/AIDS prevention and intervention*. Los Angeles, California: Lifetech Publication.

King, L.M. and Dixon, V. (Eds.) (1976). *African philosophy: Assumptions and paradigms in research on Black persons*. California, LA: Fanon Center Publications.

King, L.M. and Fluker, W.E. (1999). *The Capacity of African American churches to serve at-risk youth: a ford foundation study report*.

King, L.M. and Nobles, W. (1996). *Science, culture, church, and community: An authentic prevention model for non-insulin dependent diabetes in African American women*. Atlanta, GA.: Center for Disease Control, USDHHS.

King, L.M. and Nobles, W. (2000). *Developing the cultural perspective to guide evaluation of HIV/AIDS programs in African American communities*. SAMSA, Washington, DC. SAMSA

Kuhn, T. (1962). *The structure of scientific revolution*. Chicago: Chicago University Press.

Maddux, James E. (1993). *Social cognitive models of health and exercise behavior: an introduction and review of conceptual issues.* Special Issue: The application of social psychological theories to health and exercise.

Nijhuis, H.G. and Van der Maesen, L.J.G. (1994). The philosophical foundations of public health: An invitation to debate. *Journal of Epidemiology and Community Health*, 48: pp. 1–3.

Nobles, W. and King, L.M. (2000). Authentic models of intervention in the health of African Americans: A Prevention Approach, Washington, DC: SAMSA.

Ogden, Jano. (1995). Theory and the creation of the risky self. *Social Science Medicine*, 40: pp. 409–415.

Prochaska, J.O. and DiClemente, C.C. (1983). Stages and processes of self-change of smoking: Toward an integrative model. *Journal of Consulting and (Clinical Psychology)*, 51: pp. 390–395

Rothman, C. and Rice, D. (1998). Chronic care in America: A 21st century, institute for health and aging at University of California at San Francisco.

Rodgers, Wendy M., Brawley, and Lawrence R. (1993). Using both self-efficacy theory and the theory of planned behavior to discriminate adheres and dropouts from structured programs. Special Issue: The application of social psychological theories to health. *Journal of Applied Sport Psychology*, 5 (n2): pp. 195–206.

Stanton, B.F., Li, X., Ricardo, I., Galbraith, J., Feigelman, S., and Kaljee, L. (1996). A randomized, controlled effectiveness trial of an AIDS prevention program for low-income African-American youths. *Archives of Pediatrics and Adolescent Medicine*. Apr, 150(4): pp. 363–372.

Stein, H. (1972). Medical anthropology and the depths of human experience: contributions from psychoanalytic anthropology. *Medical Anthropology*, 14: pp. 53–75.

Stern and Steven. (1992) The opposing currents technique: For eating disorders and other false-self problems. *Contemporary Psychoanalysis*, 28(4): pp. 594–615.

Terris, M. (1983). The complex tasks of the second epidemiological revolution: The Joseph W. Mountin lecture. *Journal of Public Health Policy*, 4: pp. 8–24.

Weinstein, N.D., Rothman, A.J., and Sutton, S.R. (1998). Stage theories of health behavior; conceptual and methodological issues. *Health Psychology*, 17(n3): pp. 290–299.

Williams, D. (1990). Socioeconomic differentials in health: A review and redirection. *Social Psychology Quarterly*, 53: pp. 81–99.

Williams, R.B., Boles, M., and Johnson, R.E. (1998). A patient-initiated system for preventive health care. A randomized trial in community-based primary care practices. *Archives of Family Medicine*. July–Aug. 7(4): pp. 338–345.

Chapter **8**

The Preparation and Scope of Practice for Future Advanced Public Health Practitioners in Doctoral Programs

RENA G. BOSS-VICTORIA

Introduction

Like many aspects of American society, health care delivery is changing, influenced by political and economic pressures, new technologies, and shifting social attitudes and values. Consequently, the practice of public health practitioners must evolve based on needs and the realities of day-to-day practice in primary care and placed-based settings. Efforts to devise effective programs, strategies, and initiatives for health promotion and prevention of diseases and injuries have emerged rapidly with the creation of new opportunities to extend best-practice successes. In this light, public health, primary health care, and community-based care have experienced a renaissance in this country in the 1990's.

The Problem

Over the last fifty or sixty years, a vast body of knowledge has accumulated on health problems and health disparities in populations, their causes and prevention (epidemiology), and the management of their treatment when prevention has failed (health administration). Yet today the professional doctorate in Public Health does not begin to take proper advantage of the basic background in health and behavioral science as the preparation for a much greater social role for health improvement and behavioral change in urban African-American communities (Bryor, 1990). A much broader type of professional doctorate in Public Health is needed to support community-based practice, specifically in urban higher risk communities. The genuine, professional Doctor of Public Health that the world needs does not now exist. The schools and programs of public health around the world have become disseminators of valuable knowledge, but for many reasons their doctoral-level programs have followed the Ph.D. tradition: to prepare scholars for research and teaching, rather than preparing health leaders and practitioners for community service.

The Need for a New Metaphor for Advanced
Public Health Practitioners

The predominant direction for the future of public health mandates a focus on the current realities of the health care context. It is important that the metaphor created for change in the role and responsibilities of public health practitioners ensures an appropriate balance between the specialty content in public health, and the shared advanced practice content of the health promotion specialist. "Health for all" is a goal as valid today as when set by the World Health Assembly in 1978 (Addy, 1996). The World Health Organization (WHO) considers health a human right, and suggests that ensuring access to health care is required to achieve this goal (Addy, 1996). Public health practitioners have a major role to play, and a responsibility for achieving the goal of "health for all". It is reasonable to expect that advanced public health practitioners in communities will continue to evolve because of societal and environmental influences, as well as the internal professional growth of the discipline of public health itself.

It is time to create a metaphor for advanced public health practitioners, one that acknowledges the strengths, contributions and individuality of this role necessary for promotion of health improvements in communities, particularly in minority and challenged urban communities experiencing overwhelming disparities in health. Such leaders must have a broad knowledge of all types of problems, and all strategies for health promotion and health services management. These leaders cannot be "super-specialists" in a single topic, no matter how profound (Roemer, 1986). Public Health must conceptualize a new paradigm built from a foundation in higher education that can advance leadership development for positions in health systems, at local, state, and national levels. Professional Doctors of Public Health are needed to provide stronger leadership in policy making, particularly at the community level. Currently, physicians or doctors of clinical medicine hold most leadership and policy positions, yet very few of them have had any training in any of the numerous subdivisions of public health (Millman, 1993).

The first graduate school of public health in the world, founded at Johns Hopkins University in 1916, was initially limited to physicians (Roemer, 1999). Today, intellectual coherence in public health advances recognition of the importance of progressive educational reform. This reform provides the "communitarian" dimension, emphasizing the importance of the role that community, social and cultural context have in education, especially for advanced preparation of public health practitioners. The necessity today is to find ways to turn public health programs into functional communities that can foster commitment, concern, validation, and successful advocacy for a human practice dimension. Professionals of public health need to maintain their emphasis on educating and improving the health of higher risk populations in urban communities. The vast body of social or public health knowledge now available can support a new metaphor for an advanced public health practitioner. Regardless of the settings or community, the following goals are relevant for public health practitioners in this new millennium:

- Improved access to health care.
- Increased interdisciplinary and intradisciplinary collaboration with the health care system.
- An expanded knowledge base for health management decision-making, including health, community, and environmental assessment.
- Experience in clinical, theoretical and practical judgment, corporate, social, and institutional policy, scholarly inquiry and leadership development.
- Increased professional autonomy with eligibility for reimbursement by various payment mechanisms.

Defining Public Health Areas of Knowledge for Advanced Practitioners

The four broad areas of knowledge of public health which are core to goal achievement are (1) tools of social analysis, (2) health and disease in populations, (3) promotion of health and prevention of disease, and (4) health care systems and their management. The scope of this knowledge is surely as broad and profound as that which constitutes a medical education, but it is vastly different in content. These broad content areas are needed for the practitioner to master principles of collaborative leadership, decision-making and risk-management, regardless of setting, health or disease population (Bryor, 1990).

Social Analysis

The social analysis tools refer to such subjects as statistical reasoning, principles of epidemiology, and methods of biostatistics, which are important for analyzing data arising from epidemiology, environmental health, biomedical, and other public health-related research in a rigorous and in-depth manner. Fundamental social and behavioral science, methods, and theories continue to evolve, mandating that their functional application to contemporary public health problems moves beyond analysis to synthesis for enhanced understanding of social and behavioral variables that affect population health. The influence of poverty, social class, gender, race, family, community, work, behavioral risks, coping and resistive resources which actively confronts diverse populations requires deep content knowledge for active engagement of future public health practitioners in community settings (Braithwaite and Taylor, 1992). The tools for social analysis are essential for quality application and interpretation of scientific data for effective practice, education, and research in diverse and multicultural communities.

Health and Disease

Schools of public health have been and remain the prime resources for education, research and application of findings in disease control, based on fundamental knowledge in health and disease. Disparities in health and the prevalence of disease in special populations require a war against the major threats of cancer, stroke, heart diseases, liver disease and other potentially lethal diseases such as HIV/AIDS, which plague urban minority communities (Braithwaite and Taylor, 1992).

Despite advances in science, medicine, and public health, in nearly all countries a gap exists between the health care services available and the actual health needs of the people, irrespective of a country's level of sociopolitical and economic development (Millman, 1993; Addy, 1996). To create a future in which it is expected and accepted that the public health practitioner should occupy top leadership roles for health improvement in communities, change needs to occur in attitudes, in educational programs, and in support structures for the community-based educational process (Shugers, 1991). The professional doctorate in public health that prepares practitioners for advanced community-based practice can affect this gap. Properly trained professionals succeed through early identification of the real world or reality-based problem, and implementation plans for resolution that address the challenge of education, environment or policy change for disease control. The community-oriented, public health practice doctorate is comparable in content and time requirements to the earned research-oriented and highly specialized doctorate currently offered in public health programs. The difference is the application to practice, and the sustained emphasis in community-based settings to realize "health for all" goals, with measurable improvements in quality of life.

Health Promotion

As health promotion gains increasing prominence, all health professions strive to develop both their role and their contribution to this facet of care. The mandates of the World Health Organization (WHO), the Ottawa Charter for Health Promotion, the priorities of the National Institute for Health, and the resultant public awareness has heightened professional attention to health (WHO, 1984, 1986a; Breslow, 1990). However, educational programs for public health have continued to encompass theoretical foundations reflecting broader definitions of health and health promotion. Health promotion, most recently, has been defined as "the process of enabling people (communities and populations) to take control over and to improve their health and health status, including the intervention strategy of 'health improvement or health enhancement', or increasing the level of good health, vitality and resilience in all people" (Labonte, 1995). Yet, prevention of disease still constitutes a large part of health promotion practice. Research, largely premised upon theoretical approaches, has not clarified appropriate professional directions. Hence, health professionals' approaches to health promotion with individuals and in communities vary according to biomedical, behavioral, and socio-environmental constructions of "health" problems (Dean, 1996).

Perspectives on the concept of health promotion and disease prevention vary considerably within and between members of health professions. This confusion about the concept produces practice tensions for many health professions. Behavioral approaches focus on lifestyle modification, coping, and adaptation; whereas, disease prevention and socio-environmental strategies are oriented toward promoting well-being, and addressing the social determinants of health. As a result, in the clinical context of practice, professionals frequently use the terms "health promotion" and "disease prevention" interchangeably (Stachtchenko and Jenicek, 1990). However, the difference is of significant value for the future public health practitioner in urban communities. The professional Doctor of Public Health should be prepared to differentiate and apply appropriate meanings for health promotion in the practice role, based on the context required for the health of the population, and of society as a whole. Consequently, it is important to examine health promotion beliefs and role performance of health professionals' educational preparation in this area of care, especially as it relates to higher risk segments of urban populations.

Research confirms that curriculum emphasis alone does not ensure the practice of health promotion within or between professions (Dean, 1990; Rubin, Sobal and Moran, 1990). There is evidence to suggest that although medical and nursing professions are exposed to a variety of learning experiences relating to health promotion practice, their competence and interest in these skills are not high (Rubin, 1990; Donoghue et al., 1990). Research on other health professionals, including dental hygienists, dieticians, and nurse-midwives, identifies that differing views of health, health promotion, or the lack of effective role models and institutional influences associated with the curriculum (which is progressively more hospital-based, illness-oriented and technology focused) contributes to these findings and outcomes. Key predictors of health promotion in professional practices, beliefs, and attitudes are professional group membership and self-efficacy (Laschinger, 1996; Mullen and Holcomb, 1990). The professional public health practitioner role orientation can sharpen the more recent concept definitions of health and health promotion. These include risk reduction, risk avoidance, and health enhancement for appropriate enhancement of self-confidence and in turn, self-efficacy. Congruent interpretation and reinforcement of values, beliefs, skills, and behaviors to refine both the theory and the practice of health promotion represent the professional education milieu of the Doctor of Public Health.

Health Care Administration

It is notable that, even in situations where extensive health care services exist, people's access to medical and preventive care is often inequitable (WHO, 1994). Using WHO's (1984) definition, health care is the "provision of services to assist an individual, group or community in increasing physical capabilities, social and personal resources, to realize aspirations and safety needs, and to change or cope with the environment". Stedman (1995) further clarified the definition by stating that health care is "services provided to individuals and communities by agents of the health services or professions for the purpose of promoting, maintaining, monitoring, and restoring health" (p. 335). President Clinton, in his 1993 address to the American Heart Association acknowledged that, because of several barriers, health care is inaccessible to many U.S. citizens, particularly minorities (Moiler, 1994). Within the comprehensive definition of health and health care by WHO, a whole society—not just the medical system—has collective responsibility to achieve health for all.

Advocates of improved health care call for refocused policies on health promotion (Addy, 1996). It is quite evident that curative medicine alone is insufficient for health (Mhatre and Debre, 1992). This view declares that health is not something that only the health provider can provide. It is enhanced by community education, consumer participation, environmental and health education, and population-based strategies to improve the quality of life (Millman, 1993). The shared advanced practice content for public health practitioners must be reflective of the theoretical perspectives, research findings, and practice tools of such diverse disciplines as psychology, sociology, anthropology, communications, nursing and marketing, all of which support foundations of health, health promotion and health care system management in community-based settings (Roemer, 1996). Thus, the future public health practitioner should be required and prepared to synthesize large and diverse literatures that contribute to and blend the behavioral and social intervention process through their unique perspective for in-depth integration into the future health care system.

In the United States, the Pew Health Professions Commission identified the competencies and education needed by future health professions. According to the Commission, educational programs should incorporate the following: (1) community health and primary care; (2) prevention and promotion of health lifestyles; (3) involvement of patients and families in decision-making; (4) the role of environment; (5) racial and cultural diversity; (6) coordination of care, ensuring cost-effectiveness, and (7) information management. The Commission concluded that little change has occurred in U.S. education for health professions, although a decade of study has produced a wealth of recommendations for change. It is clear that educators must be more active in preparing health practitioners and in shaping the values and direction of health care (Shugers, O'Neil and Bager, 1991). The advanced public health practitioner of the future must enter practice prepared at a specialized level for community-based practice, a level never before achieved in doctoral programs.

BASIC TOOLS OF SOCIAL ANALYSIS	PROMOTION OF HEALTH AND PREVENTION OF DISEASE
Historical evolution of public health	Maternal and child health services
Biostatistical techniques and analyses	Mental health services
Methods of program evaluation	Communicable disease control
Political science of health systems	Control of sexually transmitted diseases
Concepts of culture and medical anthropology	Nutritional programs
Principles of medical sociology	Dental health protection
Population and demography	Health education and behavior modification
Population sampling and surveys	Chronic non-communicable disease control
Principles of health economics	Geriatrics and rehabilitation
	Environmental sanitation and protection
	Occupational health control and safety

HEALTH AND DISEASE IN POPULATIONS	HEALTH CARE SYSTEMS AND THEIR MANAGEMENT
Major diseases in humans	The national health care system
Descriptive Epidemiology (vital and health statistics)	Health workforce development
Nutrition and malnutrition	Health facilities and their administration
Infectious diseases in populations	Drugs, medical supplies, and their logistics
Chronic disorders in populations	Health planning (population-based)
Methods of clinical diagnosis and treatment	Health insurance, HMOs, and social security
Environmental hazards	Management of health programs
Mental health and disease in populations	Records and information programs
Concept of risk and epidemiological methods	Community and intersectoral relations
Global ecology of disease	Health legislation and ethics
	Health systems research
	Budgeting, cost controls, and financing
	Comparative international health systems

Figure 22.   The major content areas of public health (adapted from Roemer, 1999).

The major content areas of public health represent approximately 43 different subject domains, and emphasize the need for professional education in public health to evolve. Professional practice roles must be clarified to cultivate the meanings for each distinct area of knowledge required (Figure 22 adapted from Roemer, 1999).

The Need for New Information Channels for Community-Based Instruction, Educational, and Behavioral Change

Expanding the role of the professional Doctor of Public Health will require the examination of current perceptions of information, and the creation of new information channels, particularly as they relate to excellence in higher education (Astin, 1985). The familiar way of understanding information is as a "something" that is exchanged or created for lecture, or in conversations that focus on knowledge transmission and how to move it along smoothly without distortions. At the simplest level, a communication situation exists whenever one person transmits a message that is received by another individual, and then acted upon by that individual (Bettinghaus, 1980). However, information is not only something; it is not just content.

A new understanding of information requires an expanded definition that conceptualizes information as a structuring dynamic—a river of intelligent energy that creates order and evolution. One can view the dual nature of information through the lens of the often-told parable of the bricklayers. One describes his job as laying bricks, the other as building a cathedral. If we see our task in the development of the scope for future public health practitioners as assembling more and more bricks (content courses) presenting the perspectives of diverse disciples, we perceive information only as a thing, as a tangible entity that builds incrementally. Figure 22 fleshes out the position of content courses, but in addition to helping students understand the subject matter; the academic program also must have other, broader goals to ensure effective applications in practice. If we develop a blueprint, the academic program becomes an ordering intelligence that influences the placement of these bricks or content courses. Then, the perception of information is one of energy, with a structuring capacity as well. In other words, the academic program provides the basic content (supporting competencies and education in social analysis, health and disease, promotion of health and health systems management) but it also must relate the functions of these parts to the working of the whole scope of practice, and to the role of the community-based practitioners for health and health improvement.

Contemplating information as a process, the formative energy behind all functions and responsibilities for quality practice, allows the possession of more and new information that can be applied by the advanced practitioner to ensure growth and evolution of the healthy community. New information on public health practice and behavioral change applications in population-based strategies is created any time information meets other information, provided there is a context to give meaning to the exchange (health improvement). There is a need to create new and disconfirming information for practice and solution testing in urban communities. The old order of thinking no longer makes sense in the context of the immediate concerns of urban communities experiencing excessive disparities in health. Public health practitioners must re-organize information into a form that deals effectively with the created worldview that emerges from the populations at risk. The directions for change highlight a dynamic and evolutionary state of communities; achievement of equilibrium is almost nonexistent.

Structures (social, economic, political, corporate) are unfolding and are creatively accommodating the inherent demands of the communities, and are no longer accepted by the population when imposed without a felt need or perceived benefit. A sense of coherence and order depends on quality informational resources rather than a structure for regulation and control. Thus, information must be freely generated for learning, rather than closely managed to limit competition or opportunities. To advance new scientific principles and processes for advanced practice development, planning, and implementation based on a community-based instruction and teaching model, the essential elements for a good higher education program of preparation must be explored for incorporation.

Teaching is being re-defined as that which is planned to promote learning (Boud, 1995). Higher education programs for professional advanced public health practice in communities must facilitate effective student learning, by whatever means. Good teaching, excellence, and innovation ensure that the essential attributes and elements for learning are inherent in the academic program curriculum and educational goals (Harvey and Knight, 1996). Effective practice will not require practitioners to learn totally new technologies to work with different cultures and urban communities. Some familiar tools are transferable, because they are workable at a basic human level. The essentially familiar dynamic elements include creativity, commitment, cohesiveness, and motivation. However, what we do need to teach for effectiveness in practice is open-mindedness about the application of technologies, and how to let advanced practice students make their own meanings of the learning experience in community-based situations. The planning for learning is practical. It is not a case or theory. It focuses on a major issue or problem that the community or population faces, and must resolve creatively in order to move forward toward public health. Tactical plans and action steps are applied through the incorporated knowledge of social and system-wide analysis of the key issues along with an understanding of multidimensional health and disease responses.

Measurable learning is achieved when the learner strikes a balance between health promotion values, purpose, and meaning of situations, and options for success, growth and evolution of the health system management practices. In this transformation, possibilities for learning matter more than limits. The future for public health practice development is entirely open, ready to be created by each experience. A new synergy is experienced that bridges the gap between the way things were (the no longer) and what-will-be (the not-yet). A new perspective on the opportunities for teaching and learning emerges for public health and a genuine expertise in advanced doctoral practice.

At the professional doctoral preparation level, the purpose and coherence of the program in respect to specific aims must provide a context that can further a broad range of learning goals (Astin, 1985). The focus is on learning in relation to the program's goals, with sensitivity to the professional student's learning experiences in the context of social and cultural factors, particularly for today's new *majority* students. This new majority of students often represents individuals who are returning to school after working for a number of years, students who are adjusting to the transition of adulthood responsibilities, and competing demands. These underrepresented students further their opportunities provided by the last three decades of open access education. Learning outcomes goals for the practitioner of public health must be framed by the view of qualities and attributes required for success at work in urban communities. New graduate hires, for example, need communication skills, skill at working in large groups, analytical ability, critical thinking, time- and self-management and self-motivation (Jones, 1996). The popular success of Covey's *Seven Habits of Highly Effective People* (1991), of Goleman's *Emotional Intelligence* (1996), and of Cooper and Sawaf's *Executive EQ* (1997) reinforces the view that success at work (and in life) is about much more than intelligence, and knowledge of academic course content. Obviously, the promotion of such skills and qualities serves the students' interest. Educating students in the discipline of public health, and for life and public or private employability, implies a systematic attempt for planning at the program level, rather than at the course level. The future will emphasize bringing the learning goals of the program, and the individual courses' contribution for a greater level of coherence and quality in practice.

Essential Elements for Quality Practice-Based Teaching and Learning

Preparation for good practice in public health requires three essential elements: caring, clarity, and commitment, the three C's of formal higher education excellence (Trigwell and Prosser, 1997). The improvement of teaching for effective learning and practice requires in-depth consideration, and institutional support for the integration of these elements into the program's organizational development. The aim is to work out collective ways of improving student learning through the promotion of a learning organization that provides an environment conducive to care, clarity and commitment to community and public health practice. Caring, in the most significant sense, refers to helping one to grow and actualize. The experience of caring for a person, an ideal, or idea represents an extension of a person, but at the same time, caring is separate from the person and considerable in its own right. Caring is essential between humans if we really believe the things we say we believe. The element of caring for effective teaching is by no means a new concept; however, it remains a challenge to education, particularly as it relates to helping that is not directly connected to courses.

Caring, in the context of higher education excellence for advanced practice includes helping students with ongoing struggles toward competence, managing emotions, becoming autonomous, establishing identity, clarifying purpose, and developing integrity and confidence. In the preparation of the best and the brightest for public health practice, critical periods must be acknowledged. There are optimal times for the formation of primary social attachment, and for certain kinds of learning. This action learning may or may not be related to course content. Indeed, its significance is based more in the behavioral processes of supporting personality development that is crucial for health care professionals. Anyone who is preparing to work in a people and community-oriented field such as public health must utilize varying degrees of insights gained from modeling, even sometimes without realizing it. Excellence in teaching is expected to model and profile the element of caring. The task is appreciating the total human in the teaching and learning environment, to promote "full functioning" of public health practitioners, that is, actualization of latent capacities and potentialities for advancing caring in communities.

Programs need to develop a broad vision of student learning which is supported by face-to-face work in communities, learning tasks, and assessment arrangements to transform the emphasis to the practice realm (Hounsell, 1997). The program goals for quality practice must be given status by being reflected in the arrangement for assessing students' achievement, with higher levels of new information generation and clarity. The essential element of clarity refers to plainness of meaning and understanding. Certain concepts lend themselves more to succinct definitions than do others, which require the cognitive thinking process for ordering, classifying, and valuing new phenomena as they are encountered, including the emerging feeling of "self." The search for clarity allows the development of capacities for framing analytical, logical, evaluative thought processes for ordering things that can be quantified. Accurately understanding relational concepts, and formulating highly personalized explanations of societal phenomena to render clarity for rational decisions with predictable outcomes, enables personal-professional growth for advanced practice. Just as it is important to develop relevance and meaning for cognitive clarity, so is it important to recognize barriers to understanding for positive, meaningful learning to occur. Since public health care professionals are faced with heavy cultural, social, and human issues in community life, it is essential for students and faculty to learn to appreciate the frame of reference of others.

The element of clarity requires a shift away from the view that relevant meaning can be achieved by interpersonal distance, that is, acquired only through the sterile curriculum or stated objectives of the course. Trust and reality are interpersonal skills that advance the desired clarity for effective learning. These skills are actualized by practice, practice, and more practice in real communities with real people. In practice, students encounter situations that are not contrived, and have an opportunity to check themselves and their reflective meanings of concepts with professionals and faculty. This, in turn, fosters mutual respect, confidence, and competence. Hashing out the meaning and process for clarity is important for the preparation of the advanced practitioner concerned with understanding human behavior. He or she needs closeness and feedback from those who are perceived as models of the profession to support the experience of growth, change, and learning. Through this process, the student learns to adapt evaluative realities of situations for appropriate meanings, especially in culturally diverse urban communities.

Finally, the element of commitment refers to the passion for the work itself, or more directly, the activity that comes from the heart on behalf of another. Commitment in action for the advanced public health practitioner advances skills of advocacy, which involve genuine concern for a humane goal or cause, with assertive action to accomplish the goal, as well as an attitude that the best care for the other will be obtained at both the individual and the framework, the term of commitment reveals system level. In utilizing an advocacy model a more active meaning, defining the order of priorities for practice in urban diverse communities. Traditionally, within informal situations and, unfortunately, within many formalized public health care situations, community care encounter processes are often obtained only after someone specifically asks or demands. In addition, in the public health practice situation, the community care encounter may not be tied to a goal that is concerned with ultimate welfare. Commitment, however, along with its specific meaning, requires an involvement of active advocacy. The critical evaluation of attitudes and beliefs about what one needs to know for appropriate action on behalf of others facilitates problem-solving, consumer interest, or both.

The element of commitment calls for the advanced public health practitioner to define realistic and responsible goals. A critical ingredient for commitment development is empathy, getting at how the other perceives the world in the here-and-now. Although it is not quite so easy as the statement implies, advanced public health practitioners must learn to incorporate the values placed on both scientific know-how and the subjective, personalized experience of the community or population. Through a process of defining and evaluating with the community the care encounter situation, the totality of the experience promotes empathy, and ultimately, commitment in action. Commitment, within this framework of thinking, grows within the public health practitioner. It is a call to action that is adaptable to the special characteristics of diverse populations and communities, with particular applicability for providing care in urban settings. Commitment that involves advocacy for the community's interest and welfare allows practitioners to become activists, in that they attempt to do something in response to their growing awareness of what affects people positively or negatively in public health.

Utility beyond Agency Walls: Community-Based Practitioners in Public Health

The newly proposed public health practitioner program goal to prepare the professional Doctor of Public Health must incorporate a human care perspective to support change in health care systems and communities. Schools and programs of public health have an essential role in creating a renewed vision of learning communities for organizational change, and enhancing the teaching that supports it. Concepts such as involvement in learning, collaborative learning, distributed learning and assessment-as-learning have provided new definitions of learning in higher education. However, within the discipline of public health, who learners are—and the practical preparation for learning—is continually evolving for advanced practice in urban community-based settings. To shape scholarship for effective public health practice, new pathways must be developed, from inquiry for meaning to reflective, or deep, learning for advanced application.

Measurement of desired program goals, objectives or outcomes, competencies for learning, and assessment of effective learning are stated expectations of most accrediting agencies. Objectives are defined by the Liaison Committee on Medical Education in the Guide to the Institutional Self-Study as quantified outcomes, usually expressed in terms of behaviors, that students should acquire—learning. Therefore, the review and critique of actual measures that may be selected as realistic and appropriate expectations for advanced public health practitioners of higher education programs are required. In 1997, general attributes that might be promoted by higher education programs were defined, based on work done at the UK Quality Assurance Agency. These outcomes owed much to employers' views of the qualities they look for in new graduate hires, and defined the nature of good teaching as that which encourages such outcomes (HEQC, 1997). Figure 23 presents the attributes in cells, which are loosely grouped under four headings.

It is not expected that any higher education program would cover all of the goals shown in the cells. However, most definitely, the advanced public health program designed for community-based practice learning can select a specific array of the goals to ensure that they are promoted, and that evidence of students' achievement with respect to those selected goals can be produced for quality evaluation of aims in urban community advanced practice. Learning goals need to be explicit and plain to all stakeholders in higher education.

The learning goals for Doctors of Public Health, in order to advance community-based practice in diverse urban settings and populations, matter, and demand planning to achieve changes and create excellence in performance. The complex skills and qualities for development in advanced public health professionals require these learners to have plenty of practice in applying them in different contexts. This new model curriculum, with learning, teaching, and assessment, supports a more interventionist approach to the preparation of future advanced practitioners for public health. It advances distinctive leadership

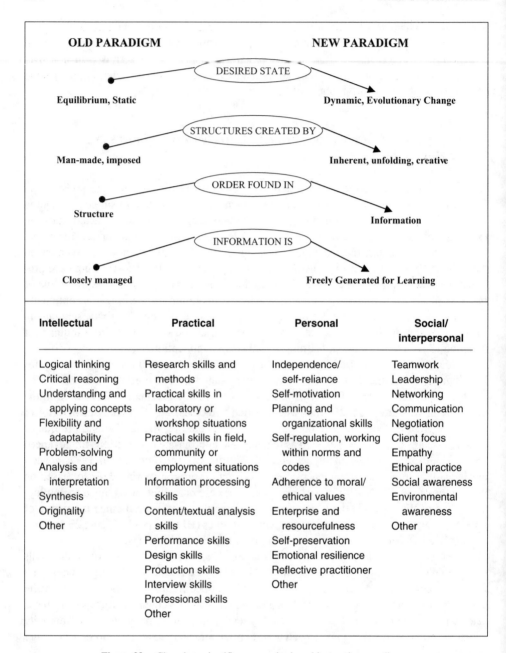

Figure 23. Changing scientific community-based instruction paradigms.

capabilities, plans for academic organizational teaching culture change, and advocates the redesign of learning to facilitate new imperatives in public health. The nature and needs of urban communities are changing, and advanced public health practitioners must be prepared to meet the direct challenge for systemic responses to systemic problems in populations in need of care.

References

Aday, L.A. and Anderson, R. (1992). Cultural impact of health—care access: Challenges for improving the health of African Americans. *Journal of Community Health Nursing;* 9(3); pp. 61–169.

Addy, J.A. (1996). Issues of access: What is going on in health care? *Nursing Economics*: 14(5): pp. 299–302.

Astin, A. (1985). *Achieving Educational Excellence: A Critical Assessment of Priorities and Practices in Higher Education*. San Francisco: Jossey Bass.

Bergquist, W.H. (1993). *The Four Cultures of The Academy*. San Francisco: Jossey Bass.

Bettinghaus, E. (1980). *Persuasive Communication*. Third Edition. New York: Holt, Richard and Winston.

Boud, D. (1995). Assessment and Learning: Contradictory or complementary? In P.T. Knight (Ed.). *Assessment for Learning in Higher Education*. London: Kogan Page.

Braithwaite, R. and Taylor, S. (1992) (Eds.) *Health Issues in The Black Community*. San Francisco, California: Jossey Bass.

Breslow L. (1990). A Health Promotion Primer for The 1990s. *Health Affairs*, Summer: pp. 6–21.

Bryor, E.L. (1990). *Scholarship Reconsidered: Priorities of the Professorate*. Princeton, N.J.: The Carnegie Foundation for the Advancement of Teaching.

Caidwell, J.C. (1993). Health transition: The cultural, social, and behavioral determination of health in the Third World. *Social Science Medicine*, 36: pp. 125–135.

Cooper, R. and Sawaf, A. (1997). *Executive EQ*. London: Orion Business Books. Covey, S. (1990). *Seven Habits of Highly Effective People*. New York: Fireside Books.

Dean, K. (1996). Using theory to guide policy relevant health promotion research. *Health Promotion International*, 11(1): pp. 19–26.

Donoghue, J., Duffield C., Pelletier, D., and Adams, A. (1990). Health promotion as a nursing function: Perceptions held by university students of nursing. *International Journal of Nursing Students*, 27(1): pp. 51–60.

Goldman, D. (1996). *Emotional Intelligence*, London: Bloomsbury.

Hounsell, D. Understanding teaching and teaching for understanding. In F. Marton, D. Hounsell and N. Entwistle (Eds.) *The Experience of Learning*, Second Edition. Edinburgh: Scottish Academic Press.

Harvey, L. and Knight, P. (1996). *Transforming Higher Education*. Buckingham: Society for Research in Higher Education and the Open University Press. Institute of Medicine (1988). *The Future of Public Health*, Washington, DC. National Academy Press.

Jones, E.A. (1996). National and state policies affecting learning expectations. In E.A. Jones (Ed.). *Preparing Competent College Graduates: Setting New and Higher Expectations in Student Learning*, (pp.7–17). San Francisco: Jossey-Bass.

Labonte, R. (1995). Population health and health promotion: What do they have to say to each other? *Canadian Journal of Public Health*, 11(1): 19–26.

Laschinger, H.K.S. (1996). Undergraduate Nursing Students: Health Promotion, Counseling, and Self-Efficacy. *Journal of Advanced Nursing*, 24: pp. 1–6.

Mhatre, S.L. and Deber, R.B. (1992). From Equal Access to the Health Care to Equitable Access to Health: Review of Canadian Provincial Health Commissions and Reports.

Millman, M. (Ed.) (1993). *Access to Health Care in America*. Washington, D.C.: Institute of Medicine

Mullen, P. and Holcomb, J. (1990). Selected predictors of health promotion Counseling by three groups of allied health professionals. *American Journal of Prevention Medicine*, 6(3): pp. 153–160.

Roemer, M.I. (1986). The need for professional doctors of public health. *Public Health Reports*, (161): pp. 21–29.

Roemer, M.I. (1999). Genuine professional doctor of public health the world needs. *Image: Journal of Nursing Scholarship*, (31)1: pp. 43–44.

Rubin, J.D., Sobal, J., and Moran, M. (1990). Health promotion beliefs and practices of fourth-year medicine students. *American Journal of Prevention Medicine*, (2): pp. 106–111.

Shugars, D.A., O'Neil, E.H., and Bader, J.D. (1991). *Healthy America: Pracitioners for 2005, an agenda for action for U.S. health professional schools*, Francisco, CA.: The PEW Health Professions Commission.

Stachtuchenko, S. and Jenicek, J. (1990). Conceptual differences between prevention and health promotion. Research implications for community health programs. *Canadian Journal of Public Health*, 81(1): pp. 53–59.

Stedman's Medical Dictionary (24th ed.) (1995). Baltimore, MD: Williams and Wilkins. Timmreck, T.C. (1987). *Dictionary of health services management* (2nd ed.). Owings Mills, MD: National Health Publishing.

Trigwell, K. and Ptrosser, M. (1997). Toward an understanding of individual acts of teaching and learning. *Higher Education Research and Development*, 16(2): pp. 241–252.

Weisbond, M. (1992). *Discovering Common Ground*. San Francisco, Berrett-Koehler Publisher.

World Health Organization (WHO). (1962). *Ottawa Charter for Health Promotion*, Ottawa: Canadian Public Health Association.

World Health Organization (WHO). (1986b). *Health promotion: A discussion document on the concept and principles*. In *Health Promotion*, Geneva World Health Organization, 1: 73–76.

World Health Organization (WHO). (1996). *Nursing Practice*. Report of a WHO Expert Committee. WHO Technical Report Series 860. Geneva, Switzerland.

Chapter **9**

The Social Context for Faith and Health

RUEBEN C. WARREN, HAROLD C.J. LOCKETT, AND ADRIAN A. ZULFIQAR

Assuring health is a major endeavor in most nations. Even when individuals and/or groups within a country cannot or have not prioritized healthy living, policy makers and health professionals attempt to maintain a reasonable standard of health for all. Assuring health is a major endeavor in most nations when individuals and/or groups prioritize health for all of their constituents. Conceptually, the goal has been to enhance physical, social, and psychological well-being and quality of life of the people who live within a country's geographical boundaries. In fact, the World Health Organization (WHO), which is a global health body, has organized nations throughout the world to collectively assure a reasonable standard of health for all (Roemer, 1976).

The World Health Organization defines health as the physical, social and psychological well-being of the individual, and not just the absence of disease (Hellberg and Maakela, 1994). Assuring physical well-being by preventing disease, disability, dysfunction, and premature death has been the primary focus of modern medical care. However, secondary social and psychological factors have also been recognized as having major influences on general health status (De La Carcela and Chin, 1998). Public health practice and departments of community and preventive medicine and dentistry have fully recognized social and behavioral factors as well as the relevant sciences associated with these factors in the health and health care paradigm (Giorgi, 1974).

While WHO has clearly defined health, a more broadened description of the perimeters of health may prove helpful. In that regard, health may be described as a relationship, a synergistic interplay between the physical, social, psychological, and spiritual elements that create the well-being of individuals and/or groups in their physical and social environment (Warren, 1999). This description surpasses the WHO definition by including the constructs of the group, spirituality, and the physical and social environment. These elements are important for all communities, but particularly for communities of color, for several reasons.

To begin with, health is a dynamic interface, a relationship between one's self and other components of society. Secondly, the group dynamic is important because it is unlikely that any health delivery system will be effective if the individual is isolated from the group. The group has an underestimated influence on an individual's decision making about health and health care issues. People seldom become ill without their family, friends or others whom they trust becoming aware and involved. They often seek advice about cause and treatment from their families and friends prior to seeking professional care. Thirdly, the role of spirituality in health and health care is increasingly recognized by the public health community to help explain why different groups with similar illnesses and treatments have very different outcomes.

Several authors suggest these so-called "incurable disorders" have been eliminated by belief, will, and faith. These phenomena, sometimes labeled spontaneous remissions, fall within the context of metaphysics, and embrace spiritual well-being (Chopra, 1989). Dismissing, ignoring, or deriding as unscientific the spiritual dimensions of diverse populations, especially people of color, is often counter-productive. To not recognize where spiritual traditions and psychological conditions often interface serves only to alienate those in need, and promotes under-utilization of services available, or worse, we cure the disease but the patient dies.

Lastly, treating a particular condition without placing it in the context of the larger environment is shortsighted and wasteful. For example, the physical and social environments are linked to several health disorders, which must be recognized if prevention or effective cures are expected. Lead has been implicated in learning disorders and anti-social behavior, such as violence (Needlemen, 1990). Mercury has been linked to neurological and reproductive disorders (Lybarger, Spengler and DeRosa, 1993). So, for health providers to concern themselves with patient symptoms, diagnosis and treatment without identifying the environmental editogy is quite myopic. Health providers unknowingly may be ignoring the greater problems of their patients, who may be living in homes with lead-based paint, or consuming large amounts of mercury-polluted fish. Moreover, they clearly are not embracing a holistic approach to health care, and the resulting treatment will undoubtedly be short-lived, at best.

Physicians as early as 2500 BC clearly understood the relationship between physical, social, psychological, spiritual well-being and health. Many of these early Egyptian physicians were also priests. They knew that influencing human behavior and social circumstances was key to maintaining one's physical health (Rogers, 1947).

Within this expanded definition of health, several important dimensions are worthy of special attention. To be physically healthy, body structures must be maintained in an optimal anatomical and physiological state. Diseases must be eliminated as much as possible, and body structures must be examined regularly to prevent dysfunction. Socially, body structures and functions must allow the individual to thrive in this complex postmodern society (i.e., employment and school). Therefore, support systems, including the health delivery system, need to be holistic. Unfortunately, seldom are these systems comprehensive enough to address social conditions, leaving many groups underserved.

Being physically healthy reduces many of the barriers that prevent people from reaching their life goals (McCord and Freman, 1990). Psychologically, the lack of a healthy body is a barrier to positive self-esteem and psychological development. Poor physical appearance and limited mobility and agility can, and often do, lead to negative self-images, lack of self-confidence, and self-defeating behaviors (Chunn and Dunston, 1983). Spiritual well-being adds meaning and purpose to life, thus serves as the foundation for maintaining a sustained quality of life (Taylor, 1993).

Historically, global threats to health have been grouped into three basic categories: infectious disease threats, chronic disease threats, and occupational and environmental disease threats (American Journal of Public Health, 1983). For example, over a century ago, William Alison, Professor of Medical Jurisprudence at Edinburgh University, described the association between poverty and infectious diseases. His experience with epidemic typhus and relapsing fever in 1827, and the Cholera Epidemic of 1831 confirmed his observations. The causes of death in these epidemics were infectious diseases (Sigerist, 1940). In 1826, Louis Rene Villerme, a French scientist, described incredible living conditions that caused premature death, which again were associated with infectious diseases. Even John Snow's classic work on cholera describes the various ways in which poverty and destitution influenced the causative agents to the host and environment (Terris, 1992). The focus was to look for infectious agents. Henry E. Sigerist (Siegerist, 1946), the great medical historian, stated that "Health is promoted by providing a decent standard of living, good labor conditions, education, physical exercise, culture, and means of rest and recreation." Their attention was on infectious diseases, and rightly so. This pattern also existed in the United States.

However, in more recent years, chronic diseases have replaced infectious diseases as the leading cause of death, particularly in the United States. Heart disease, cancer, and diabetes have been leading causes of morbidity and mortality within all race/ethnic groups for many years (National Center for Health Statistics, 1998). The World Health Organization recently reported that by the year 2020 chronic diseases would account for 70% of deaths throughout most of the world (Ruttier, 1998). Unfortunately, many chronic diseases have no permanent cure; therefore prevention is the best strategy. Ironically, the current approach to improving health is, at best, only a beginning to curing and controlling diseases, particularly chronic diseases such as heart disease, cancer, and diabetes, because these chronic diseases have no real biomedical cure. Therefore, the need to devise more effective prevention strategies for chronic diseases is an imperative. While strategies for prevention and cure of infectious diseases have accounted for major reduction in global morbidity and mortality, chronic diseases reduction will be far more expensive, difficult, and protracted.

As the third era of global health threats emerges, one finds an even more alarming trend. Occupational and environmental health threats are a mixture of biomedical and behavioral risk factors. The science necessary to address the prevention, treatment and cure of occupational and environmental related diseases and disabilities is relatively new and evolving (Cullen and Rosenstock, 1998). The behavioral, social, political, and economic uncertainties complicate this era; consequently there has been a delay in adequately addressing these threats to human health, environment and the quality of life (Johnson, Williams and Harris, 1992).

Clearly, specific populations, particularly in the United States, disproportionately suffer the burden of disease; dysfunction, disability and premature death associated with occupational and environmental health threats. As with infectious and chronic disease threats, racial/ethnic minority populations, including, African American, Hispanic/Latino, Native American and targeted Asian American and Pacific Islander subgroups, are at the greatest risk (Walker, Goddwin and Warren, 1993). Low income, undereducated and geographically isolated groups also have disproportionate health risks associated with occupational and environmental threats (Institute of Medicine, 1999). If one belongs to more than one of these groups, (i.e., low-income Latino living in rural America) a "layering effect" worsens the burden (U.S. Department of Health and Human Services, 1985). Even worse, unless the broader description of health is considered, a narrow approach to reduce the risks and promote health may be used, which will only address a portion of the health concerns.

This chapter, therefore, addresses the social context of faith and health as a theoretical framework for promoting health and improving the quality of life for individuals and groups. It attempts to provide insight into how behavioral and social sciences and other social constructs such as faith provide a critical context for improving health. The sections in this chapter include (1) synergic relationship between religion, faith and health; (2) a global overview of the concepts of religion; (3) review of the major morbidity and mortality and their social and behavior associations; (4) the religious/faith influence on health and health care; (5) health promotion strategies which focus on individual/groups behavior and (6) significance and expected outcome.

Synergistic Relationship between Religion, Faith, and Health

In attempting to address issues of health among people, particularly people of color, one must acknowledge the limited perspective of many people regarding health that limits the success of the various health interventions that have been attempted (Choi and Greenberg, 1982). What often occurs is an analysis of health status based on adverse health outcomes such as disease, disability, dysfunction, and premature death. These outcomes have usually been physical health outcomes (National Center for Health Statistics, 1998). There has been less effort to measure psychological outcomes (DeLaCarcela, Chin and Jenkins, 1998). Even less has been done to integrate social outcome measures of health, although social risk factors such as poverty, undereducation, underemployment, and poor living conditions have been associated repeatedly with excess morbidity and mortality (Terris, 1992). Spiritual influences on diseases and disabilities, though clearly associated with physical health, are seldom considered when health status is assessed (Chissell, 1993). To more effectively address health issues, all four components of health should be considered. Deepak Chopra, M.D. (Chopra, 1995) states in his tape "Creating Health" that the one's psychological and physical health and well-being are inextricably linked. He argues convincingly that people become sick because they have conditioned themselves to believe that sickness and disease are inevitable. Chopra is an endocrinologist. He provides several examples of physical illness and disease, such as hypertension and ulcers resulting from psychological stressors. He suggests that some cancers and other "incurable" disorders have been cured by belief, will and faith. Some of these "cures" are called spontaneous remission. Dr. Chopra is an East Indian physician living in the United States.

Another author, M. Scoff Peck, M.D. (Peck, 1978) is a psychiatrist. In his book *The Road Less Traveled* he writes about the power of "non-biological forces" that provide spiritual health and relief of both physical and mental disorders. Dr. Venice Bloodworth, (Bloodworth, 1979) a psychologist, in her text "Key to Yourself" explores many thoughts about the conscious, subconscious and universal mind as tools for health and well being. All of these authors are well-versed in the biomedical sciences, and they all suggest that health is abundant, and that the ingredients for maintaining health are plentiful and accessible in nature—good food, exercise, good relationships, laughter, rest and happiness, to name a few.

John Chissell (1993), a family physician, explores African concepts of faith and health in his book entitled *Pyramids of Power*. He outlines several components related to total well-being for both the individual and the group. He supports the idea that an expanded description of health will clearly result in a broader set of risk factors and a broader array of interventions.

One's ability to take personal responsibility for his or her health is in part, determined by the ability to control those factors that influence their life circumstances. This is often referred to as "locus of control." One's locus of control will ultimately determine an individual's perception of his/her ability to influence the factors that control life, health and well-being (Kerting, 1973). Within the broader description of health there are several areas that can be controlled both at the individual and group level. For the most part, this control is accomplished through belief systems, religious practices, and faith. However, even before exploring these possible social/behavior controls, a review of the religion/faith interface throughout history must be undertaken.

A Global Overview of the Concepts of Religion

The role of priest as a prerequisite to becoming a physician is well documented in ancient Egyptian kingdoms (Te Velde, 1995). Anthropological studies of hunter-gather societies document that most activity surrounding the art of healing also includes the notion of faith in some external, eternal source of power that would allow health to be regained (Schrire, 1984). For the majority of human beings, the expression of faith is equated with religion (Al-Faruqi, 1974). However, the concept of faith does not require religion. Human beings have the capacity of having faith in something while not prescribing to a particular religion. Agnostics, for example, may denounce a particular religious belief, but do not always reject the concept of faith. Although faith and religion are not synonymous, exploring of the connection between faith and health must begin with greater insight into various religious ideologies. Even when faith and religion are not used interchangeably, one cannot understand faith without first reviewing the major religious systems in different parts of the world.

There are numerous religions throughout the world that can be found in virtually every corner of the globe. The most common are Christianity (Protestants and Catholics combined), Islam, Buddhism, and Hinduism (Jainism and Sikhism included), respectively. Other religions with significant numbers include Judaism, Taoism, and what can be referred to as African traditional religions. Religions such as Zorastianism, Bahism, and Native American spirituality, while smaller in numbers, still thrive throughout the world. Based on their size, for the purposes of this chapter, the five major religions of Christianity, Islam, Judaism, Hinduism and Buddhism will be explored (Al-Faruqi, 1974). Excluding other religions and religious systems, however, does not diminish their importance, value or significance.

Amidst the tenets of religions, there are some spiritual notions for which there exist no set definitions, even after centuries of scholarly study and debate (Mahoney, 1999). The foundation of some religious beliefs is based on the concept of a soul, which provides definition to the experience of faith. The Christian apostle Paul states in the New Testament, "Faith is the substance of things hoped for; evidence of things unseen." Faith and spirituality are closely linked, and an important factor in spirituality is the need for the discovery of something unknown. The common unknown factor for Abrahamic religions (Judaism, Christianity and Islam, all believing that Abraham was the "father" of their faith) may be in the discovery of the "straight path" (*sirat-al-mustakeem*) or the fostering of one's relationship with God (Al-Faruqi, 1986). In Buddhism or Hinduism the essence of spirituality is more abstract and can be embodied in the discovery of self or escaping the wheel of karma. Karma is literally translated as action; there is good and bad karma. In essence, spirituality is the "way of living" that allows one to give meaning to life and purpose to one's actions (Covey, 1989).

To understand where faith originates and how spirituality is defined, one must first understand the religious traditions that dictate the understanding of these particular elements. Although there are many spiritual individuals without any particular affiliation to religion, the majority of the world's people affiliate with a particular religious creed

(Al-Faruqi, 1974) In describing several religious traditions; one discovers the emergence of faith as a common theme.

Christianity is reported to have the largest contingency of believers when compared to other religions. With this in mind, the division of Protestants and Catholics is largely irrelevant considering that even the thesis written by Martin Luther, sparking the Protestant Reformation, did not focus on the actual concept of God, but rather on human authority in the church (Chadwick, 1995). Furthermore, the various Protestant religious groups comprise significant communities in themselves. Thus, only the core Christian beliefs regarding notions of reality and God are of concern, and they are relatively consistent amidst the diversity. The doctrine of Trinity stands at the basis of Christian thought concerning God. This doctrine presents the belief that God is one, comprising three entities in the one: God, Jesus Christ, who is considered the embodiment of God on earth, and the Holy Spirit (Al-Faruqi, 1974). Central to this concept is the *one*, which serves as a reference point; an eternal being that is external to this world. The powers vested in God embody perfection as the creator of all humanity and all natural things. As creator then, God is also the director of actions on earth, thus having a plan that humans follow in the patterns of their daily lives. This God-directed plan is fundamentally important when considering the relationship of Christian believers to their health. If, God is controlling the earth, then one very easily is able to rely on the notion that God is aware of one's suffering; hence, there is some reason for it. If an individual uses spiritual reasons for their illness, they may also divide their illness between the physical realm and a greater entity at work that can ensure their health. Thus, their healing is divided between God and the doctor.

The Hebrew teaching, that man/woman is a unity of soul and body, and that neither is complete without the other, is retained in Christian thought from ancient Judaism (Al-Faruqi, 1986). This connection further suggests the influence that faith can have on the physical health of a Christian. With the soul and body connected, there are two implications. First, the soul is an entity that cannot be grasped, since its existence is abstract in itself. Hence, this abstract notion has an effect on the total well-being of the individual. Second, the soul is directly connected to the unseen and unknown; thus, one's belief in the unknown and unseen is directly related to the well-being of the soul. Hence, since the soul is connected to the body, then the well-being of the soul naturally affects the body.

Islam has the second largest religious following in the world (Buchsbaum, 1993). Islam uses the Koran as its scripture, believing that this was the direct revelation of God to the prophet Muhammad. The fundamental belief of Islam is the declaration of faith (*shahada* in Arabic) that states: "There is no God, but Allah, and Muhammad is the messenger of Allah." (Al-Faruqi, 1982) For this chapter the second part of this declaration is not of particular significance because Muhammad does not have a role, like Jesus for Christians, where he is involved in the actual understanding of God. Alternatively, the conception of oneness or unity of God known as *tawhid* is the foundation upon which the rest of Islamic belief rests. Tawhid is a negation of all worship besides God (Allah) and an affirmation of the supreme nature of God. It also determines much of the consciousness of the Muslim about his or her health (Al-Faruqi, 1982). The *shahada* itself is part of the five pillars in Islam. The other four pillars are fasting, pilgrimage, prayer and charity (these are rough translations of the Arabic). Allah, or God, is seen as residing outside of this world, but being as close to a believer as the believer's "jugular vein." (Ali) Therefore, Allah is everywhere, and ever watchful of all that happens on earth. Like the God of Christianity, Allah also is the creator and the planner of all that goes on. There is a strong belief in the afterlife; thus there are constant references in the Koran on the temporary nature of the existence on earth. This belief pattern among Muslims allows them to cope with concepts of death and dying more easily. The belief is that all things are in subservience to God, hence the "sun sets and rises at prescribed times always from the East to the West, and the moon goes through a consistent pattern of waxing and waning under Allah's control." (Saleem)

> In the alternation of night and day; in the ships that sail the ocean with cargoes benefi-cial; in the water, Allah sends down from the clouds and with which He revives the dead earth and with which He dispersed over it all kinds of animals; in the movement of winds and in the clouds that are driven between the earth and the sky surely are signs for men of understanding. (Ali)

The consistency of life not only provides a sign of God's existence, but also further that God has instructed reality to follow a pattern according to his design. Thus, any ill-ness that occurs is to be considered for one's own benefit, although it may not seem that way at the time. The benefit is considered to be a part of life for Muslims. However, the believer is reassured that it will not be a burden that they cannot bear. "No burden do we place on any soul, but that which it can bear." (Ali)

Health assurances for the Muslim are based on several factors that serve to increase their well-being. First, the believer is assured that this life is temporary so everything in this life is simply a test that will determine their place in the next life. Thus, a believer accepts the notion of fate. Second, they believe that God is working in their best interest and according to a plan that provides symmetry to the earth. Finally, they trust that a bur-den will never be too great, so no matter the difficulty, no illness is too much to endure. The practical application of these concepts to the average believer's life can be readily observed, even among the weakest believers.

Judaism is considered the first of the Abrahamic religions and has two major scrip-tures known as the Tanakh and the Talmud. The Tanakh consists of the Torah (first five books of the Old Testament), Nevi'im (the Prophetic books of Isaiah, Amos, etc.) and the Ketuvim (the Writings" including Kings, Chronicles, etc.). The Talmud contains stories, laws, debates, etc., and is composed from the Misnah and the Gemara (Cohn-Sherbock, 1999). The Jewish conception of God is very similar to that of Christianity and Islam. The God in Judaism is the creator of all that exists, and the absolute ruler of the universe. God monitors the activities of humans and he punishes evil, while rewarding good. God is also one, and nothing else can be worshiped besides God. Twice daily a prayer (Shema) is recited which affirms this belief by beginning: "Hear, Israel.' The Lord is our God, The Lord is one" (48).

God also has no body, is neither male nor female, and is omnipotent. By following the divine commandments (mitzvot), Jewish people are able to sanctify their lives and draw closer to God. Jewish people are also the chosen people, whom God has selected to fulfill his covenant. The Jewish religion regards actions as far more important than belief, and there is a belief that God has a larger plan which dictates our actions on earth (Cohn-Sherbock, 1999) Unlike the other two Abrahamic religions, Judaism does not have much dogma about the afterlife, since the primary concern is given to this life and actions here on earth. Conclusions that can be drawn from the description of Judaism are somewhat similar to both Christianity and Islam. The belief in the power of God allows a Jewish per-son to recognize a greater plan and reinforces the belief that God is looking out for his/her betterment. Jewish people are also assured that they are the "chosen people" and hence they have nothing to fear from God, since he is always just. The transmission of hope for a Jewish person resides solely with God.

Hinduism provides a separation from the systems of religion known as Abrahamic. Hinduism came from no one founder, and is a collection of sacred writings that do not have rules, as we know them (Al-Faruqi, 1974). The various expressions of Hindu religion vary from the region where one lives, to the specific city where one is born. Each Hindu is born as part of a caste (jati) that prescribes his or her responsibilities in this life. Hindis are all working within the cycle of reincarnation in order to break the cycle. The concept of God or gods falls into what has been labeled as "passive monotheism". This term is generally understood to mean a fleeting worship of one main deity at one time (Al-Faruqi, 1951). Hence, there may be a pantheon of gods, but the Hindu may choose specific ones to give special reverence on any particular day. For instance, if it is raining and they do not want rain, then the rain god (or the equivalent) would be referenced. There are various places where the Lord of the gods is mentioned, however there are several gods that have been designated the "creator of creatures." There is also a widespread belief in the pre-planned nature of life. Certain individuals on earth are even vested with powers to predict and tell the future of people's lives. This belief creates a mentality in individuals that puts them at ease with their current situation since it could not have been avoided, or otherwise, would go against God's plan and challenge God's uniqueness. The transmission of belief thus is placed upon a variety of gods who are seen as saviors for specific needs, while the pre-determined nature of life allows acceptance of one's condition.

Buddhism is similar to Hinduism in many ways, although Buddha himself is supposed to have refuted Hinduism and its lifestyle. Buddha is the main figurehead of Buddhism. The Buddhist belief is very much focused on relieving oneself of the cycle of rebirth, just as in Hinduism, but it is very much against all extreme measures to attain this relief (Keown, 1996). A middle course is advocated in all circumstances, known as, "the Middle Path". The ultimate goal in life is to obtain nirvana, a point of enlightenment. The Buddha described four steps necessary for enlightenment to occur known as the Noble Truths. The first of the truths is that suffering exists, and the very fact of living implies suffering. The second truth is that the cause and/or origin of suffering is the time devoted to conquering one's desires (tanha). The third truth advises how to end suffering—by eliminating all desires and wants. The fourth and final truth is the cessation of suffering, and must follow the Noble Eightfold Path (Keown, 1996). The eight aspects of the Buddha when describing this path were: right views, right conduct, right speech, right aims, right effort, right mindfulness, and right meditation. Buddha did not deny the existence of God, but in fact, rendered God useless in the broader picture of attempting to obtain enlightenment. The focus is on understanding one's present condition before venturing off into other avenues. This framework is significant for all Buddhists who are instilled with a particular mentality that allows a better understanding of the world. The Buddhist understands first that the self must be kept pure and therefore considers preservation of his or her health an important matter. Hence, health promotion and disease prevention are measures, which are very effective with Buddhists. Furthermore, understanding is still focused on an eternal, external entity of the true or ideal self. The attainment of this ideal self is the purpose of the believer's life in order that he or she may achieve enlightenment (Healey, 1997).

The concepts of religion reviewed are a fundamental part of the upbringing and thought pattern instilled into the believers of all of the religions described. Believers are taught these principles at an early age. These believers are then cultured with the basic concepts of their own faiths. Even if their actions are not in accordance with the religion, their mindset is consistent with their belief.

With a general review of some of the larger religions, it is important to now consider the implications of their convergence. The working hypothesis is that there is a point where religions broadly converge. At this point of convergence is a consistent element called faith, and faith can be found in both religious and non-religious groups. Understanding the growing number of religions in the world, will allow one to identify his or her converging faiths. Inherently, it seems that all religions, even the ones newly formed, rely on some notion or entity that is external to the believers, as they know themselves. Every religion must rely on something that is relatively unknown. John Hicks extracts certain parts of various scriptures to show the convergence on what he refers to as the "Ultimate Reality or the Real" (Asian, 1998).

From Judaism:
"With a great love have you loved us, O Lord our God and with exceeding compassion. You pitied us. Our Father and King."

From Islam:
"Praise be to God, Lord of creation, Source of all livelihood, who orders the morning Lord of majesty and honor, of grace and beneficence."

From Sikhism:
"There is but one God. He is all that is. He is the Creator of all things and He is all pervasive."

From Hinduism:
"Then I their name shall magnify, And tell their praise abroad, For very love and gladness I shall dance before my God."

For Hick, then, the notion of convergence relies on the logic that if there are a variety of believers out there who are turning their focus towards a transcendent entity, could it be that this entity is one Reality? In this thinking, the God that is worshiped by Christians must also be that of Muslims, Jews, Sikhs and certain Hindus, because each has an equal claim to truly worshiping God. Furthermore, the "infinite conceptions of Being-Consciousness-Bliss (Satchitananda)" in Hinduism or the "ineffable cosmic Buddha nature (Dharmakaya) of some forms of Buddhism all relate to the 'theistic streams' of this personal religious presence" (Hicks and Hebblethwaite, 1981).

Sewed Hossein Nasr saw the same concept of religious pluralism as the "different manifestations of the immutable everlasting truth." According to Nasr, at the heart of every religion there is a *religion perennis* that contains a "doctrine regarding the nature of reality and a method which prescribes the attainment of Reality as such." Each religion has a variety of prescriptions; however, the ultimate goal and purpose remain the same, universally (Asian, 1998).

Although Hicks and Nasr approach religious convergence from two different perspectives, the essence of both their thoughts is the same. It is possible to find common threads within the religions of the world, because of the consistent characteristics that go into formulating a religion. This is vital when understanding the interplay of religious belief and health. The connection of mind and body is becoming more apparent as health researchers discover the undeniable connection between a patient's psychological state and their physical health. Outside the realm of religion, when the convergence of faith occurs, spirituality assumes an important role. Spirituality is defined by the core essence of each of the religions, and the reliance on the notion of reality or immutable truth. Spirituality may not necessarily be based on dogmatic rules, but will find its expression in the fundamental beliefs of different religions, those beliefs that are largely part of the journey that each religion asks its believers to take. Hence, the spirituality of the Buddhists' search for enlightenment is similar to the Muslims' quest to embody the "way of the prophets" (*sunnah*). Spirituality is then a positive reinforcement of the ideals and values that are universally a part of faith. The Hindu scripture known as the Bhagavad Gita states:

> Howsoever men may approach me, even so do I accept them; for on all sides whatever path they may choose is mine. (Hick and Hebblethwaite, 1981)

Similarly, the Persian poet, Jalaluddin Rumi summarizes the proposition concerning the importance and convergence of faith by stating:

> The lamps are different, but the Light is the same: it comes from Beyond. (Hick and Hebblethwaite, 1987)

In the final analysis, religions converge upon faith in something that transcends the human existence. This faith then provides the medium for a spirituality that encompasses the believers' thinking and actions. Furthermore, religion is not a necessary component for spirituality, because faith in things transcendent to one's presence can occur outside of an institutionalized religion. As Rumi has pointed out, "the lamps are the same", whether they be institutional religion or simply personal faith. The important similarity is that the light comes from "beyond."

Review of the Trends in Major Morbidity and Mortality and Their Social and Behavioral Associations

Decreases in mortality and morbidity continue as improvements and benefits of biomedical research and health care delivery reach more people. While the United States purports to have the best health care system in the world, the health of people who live in the U.S. varies considerably. Race, ethnicity, income, education, and occupation differences account for the varying health status between these groups. African Americans, Hispanic/Latinos, Native Americans, and certain subgroups of Asian American or Pacific Islander are likely to have worse health status than their non-Hispanic white counterparts. Those who are lower-income and/or under educated, or working or living in unhealthy or unsafe environment are also more likely to be sicker. These demographic factors have resulted in disproportionate health risks of disease, disability, and premature death among minorities. Even as the health threats change, the burdens of disease and risks do not change measurably for these groups (U.S. Department of Health and Human Services, 1985).

As previously indicated, health threats have changed both in magnitude and type over the years (American Journal of Public Health, 1999). Figure 24 indicates a major shift in causes of death in the United States from infectious diseases to chronic diseases. Heart diseases for example, represented 8.0% of the deaths in 1900; cancer represented 3.7%. By 1996, these two chronic diseases moved from being the 4th and 8th leading causes of deaths to being the first and second. More than 50% of the deaths in 1996 were attributed to one of these two conditions. Another example of the shifting causes of death, and measures to quantify these shifts, is the years of potential life lost (YPLL). This measure calculates premature deaths by using the years of potential lost life under 75 years of age. In 1995, 1,587.70 and 1,259.20 YPLL were lost per 100,000 people, due to cancer and

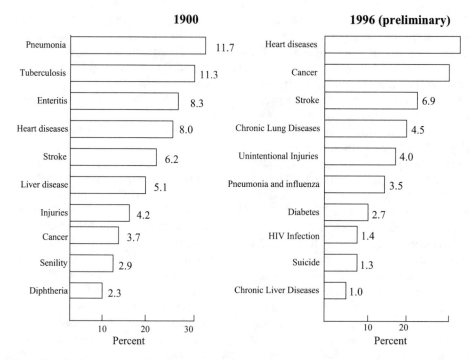

Figure 24. Ten leading causes of death as a percentage of all deaths: United States, 1900 and 1996 (*Source*: CDC, National Center for Health Statistics).

Causes of death	YPLL*	% change since 1990
Cancer	1,587.70	−7.4
Heart Disease	1,259.20	−7.6
Unintentional Injuries	1,555.50	−8.5
Intentional Injuries	842	−3.5
HIV/AIDS	570.3	55.7
Stroke	211.5	−4.3
Chronic Obstructive Pulmonary Disease	161.4	2.9
Diabetes	149.9	12.7
Liver Disease and Cirrhosis	149.7	−11.3
Pneumonia and Influenza	115.3	−10.3
All Causes (Total)	**8,128.20**	**−4.8**

*Years lost per 100,000 population under 75 years of age.

Figure 25. YPLL before age 75 by cause of death, 1995 (*Source*: CDC, National Center for Health Statistics).

heart diseases, respectively (See Figure 25). If the causes of death are shifting, strategies to identify and reduce a new set of risk factors must also be designed (U.S. Department of Health and Human Services, 1998).

Figure 26 lists the leading cause of death for women by race and Hispanic origin in 1996. Figure 27 lists the same data for men. With the exception of Asian American women, diseases of the heart and cancer ranked first and second for both genders and all race/ethnicity categories. In causes of death categories other than congenial abnormities, the risk factors for all of the causes of death in Figures 26 and 27 are behavior related. The previous examples of changes in the causes of death by gender, race and Hispanic origin consistently chronicle race and Hispanic origin as notable factors in morbidity and mortality. African Americans have had consistently higher death rates than other races and ethnic groups (Collins, Hall and Neuhaus, 1998).

Another measure used to record health status in most countries is infant mortality. Figure 28 lists infant mortality by race and Hispanic origin. Infant mortality rates have been declining for all U.S. racial and ethnic groups. However, the disparity remains constant. African Americans have the highest infant mortality rate, with 14 deaths per 1,000 live births. Native Americans have the next, with 10 deaths per 1,000 live births. Among Hispanics mothers, Puerto Ricans have the highest infant mortality rate at 8.6 deaths per 1,000 live births; Mexicans, 5.8; Cubans, 5.1 and Central and South Americans, (5.0) (MacDorman et al., 1998). African American infant mortality is related to higher rates of complicated pregnancies, adverse birth events, and higher rate of low-birth weight babies. Excess deaths among very low birth weight infants account for 62% of the racial disparity in infant mortality (Rowley, 1995). Unfortunately, all of the factors associated with infant mortality have not been identified, and the gap remains (Collins, Hall and Neuhaus, 1998).

Due to advancements in biomedical research and health care, overall health status in the United States continues to improve. At the same time, appropriate public health measures and health services have not been translated and transmitted to those in the greatest need. Consequently, the health gaps in the United States are not closing at rates commensurate with the technology that is available.

Margaret Heckler (U.S. Department of Health and Human Services, 1985), former Secretary of Health and Human Services in the Introduction to the 1985 *Report of the Secretary Task Force on Black and Minority Health*, wrote

> There was a continuing disparity in the burden of death and illness experienced by the Blacks and other minority Americans as compared to the Nation as a whole. The disparity has existed ever since accurate Federal record keeping begin more than a generation ago. And although our health charts do itemize steady gains in the health of minority Americans, the stubborn disparity remained … an affront to both our ideals and the ongoing genius of American medicine.

Some believe that the health disparity is most strongly based on income and education. However, even when income and/or education are constant, ethnic and racial differences within income and education remain. Gender, age, and geographic differences also account for the disparity of health status. Nonetheless, differences based on race and ethnicity still remain, even when these demographic variables are held constant (U.S. Department of Health and Human Services, 1985). What is clear is that ethnic and racial backgrounds are very important factors and must be considered in any strategy to improve the health of any group of people. However, much has to be done to better understand the role of race and ethnicity on health and health care delivery; a scientific inquiry and strategic plan are needed. If the health of the nation is to improve, the health of every group within the nation must improve. This is particularly true and urgent in the United States because of the rapidly changing demographics.

In reviewing health risk factors and likely interventions, social and behavioral sciences become more and more important. Victor Fuchs (1974), an economist, in his book

All Females	White	Black	Rank	Native American	Asian American	Hispanic
Heart Disease	Heart Disease	Heart Disease	1	Heart Disease	Cancer	Heart Disease
Cancer	Cancer	Cancer	2	Cancer	Heart Disease	Cancer
Cerebrovascular Disease	Cerebrovascular Disease	Cerebrovascular Disease	3	Accidents and unintentional injuries	Cerebrovascular Disease	Cerebrovascular Disease
Chronic Lung Disease	Chronic Lung Disease	Diabetes	4	Diabetes	Accidents and unintentional injuries	Diabetes
Pneumonia and influenza	Pneumonia and influenza	Accidents and unintentional injuries	5	Cerebrovascular Disease	Pneumonia and influenza	Accidents and unintentional injuries

Figure 26. Leading causes of death for women by race and Hispanic origin, 1999 (*Source*: National Center for Health Statistics, 1998; Collins, Hall and Neuhaus, *U.S. Minority Health: A Chart Book* 1999).

All Males	White	Black	Rank	Native	Asian American	Hispanic
Heart Disease	Heart Disease	Heart Disease	1	Heart Disease	Heart Disease	Heart Disease
Cancer	Cancer	Cancer	2	Accidents and unintentional injuries	Cancer	Cancer
Cerebrovascular Disease	Cerebrovascular Disease	HIV infection	3	Cancer	Cerebrovascular Disease	Accidents and unintentional injuries
Accidents and unintentional injuries	Accidents and unintentional injuries	Accidents and unintentional injuries	4	Diabetes	Accidents unintentional injuries	HIV infection
Chronic Lung Disease	Chronic Lung Disease	Homicide	5	Chronic liver disease and cirrhosis	Pneumonia and influenza	Homicide

Figure 27. Leading causes of death for men by race and Hispanic origin, 1999 (*Source:* National Center for Health Statistics, 1998; Collins, Hall and Neuhaus, *U.S. Minority Health: A Chart Book* 1999).

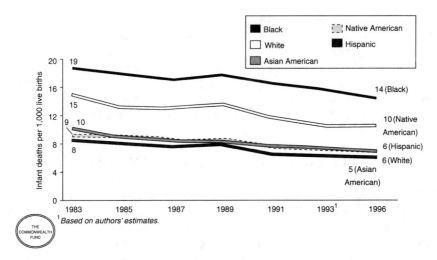

Figure 28. Infant mortality rates by race and Hispanic origin, 1983–1996 (*Source*: Council of Economic Advisers, 1998, Anderson et al., 1997, and MacDorman et al., 1998).

"Who Shall Live," writes that after a certain point, health improvements are not influenced by technology, income or education. The factors that influence health are many times beyond the control of the health delivery system. Nonetheless, there are many interventions within the public health arena and health care delivery that have proven efficiency. For example, Leavell (Leavell and Clark, 1965) in his classic approach to preventive medicine, describes three levels of prevention: primary, secondary, and tertiary. Primary prevention is effective in the absences of disease (i.e., pre-pathologic); health education, disease prevention and health protection strategies are needed, such as water, fluoridation and vaccinations. Secondary prevention is needed to eliminate or reduce diseases in the early stages. While this stage of prevention is also effective, it is not as efficacious as primary prevention. Tertiary prevention requires extensive rehabilitation and surgical procedures, which usually require more training and money. Tertiary prevention, in fact, is less effective than primary and secondary prevention in improving health. Leavell suggests that care is a continuum, from prevention to cure. However, the premise for his approach assumes that disease and illness are inevitable. Alternatively, if the assumption is that disease and premature death are not inevitable, a different paradigm may be considered. And for the purposes of this chapter, the paradigm shift proposed is from disease cure to disease prevention to health promotion. Ideally, creative health promotion interventions can be designed and implemented before diseases and disabilities occur and focused on health protections and health enhancements.

Health promotion, however, has taken on numerous definitions, and is best described by Tannahill (1985) as compromising "efforts to enhance positive health and reduce the risk of ill-health through overlapping spheres of health education, prevention and promotion." Health promotion is positive and proactive, while clearly recognizing the threats and consequences of disease, disability and premature death. Health promotion, he writes, has as a cardinal principle the empowerment of the individual and group to enhance their health and quality of life, even in the midst of disease and threats to life. Health promotion challenges the notion that "one has to get sick".

The authors of this chapter recognize the accomplishments of biomedical research and the health delivery system. Through these accomplishments—antibiotics, vaccines, fluoridation and other great improvements in public health have occurred. These solutions have come primarily through biomedical research translated into public health action. However, the impact of biomedical research on social and behavioral problems adversely effecting health is limited. Social and behavioral sciences and scientists must assume a more proactive role in public health if more improvements in health of the public are to be expected.

The Influence of Religion and Faith on Health and Health Care

Peter Berger (Berger, Berger and Kellner, 1973) in his book entitled "The Homeless Mind" writes that society is laden with high technological advancements. He refers to the modern technological society as "modernity". As advances are made in this post-modern society, challenges continue to mount related to these technical advancements, such as the Y2K Crisis. Consequently, the limitations of technology also have become more apparent.

Similar events are occurring in health care delivery. As technology continues to advance, financial and geographical access to the technology becomes more limited (Berger, Berger and Kellner, 1973). Racism, sexism, homophobia, and other discriminatory practices by providers and payers also continue to mount (Warren, 1997). Ethical issues on how and when to use the technology are also under serious debate (Berger, Berger and Kellner, 1973). A postmodern society requires policy makers to move beyond technology to find more creative ways of providing services, including health services. In fact, the health industry no longer depends solely on doctors to maintain healthy populations. More and more, the health delivery system is seeking health strategies beyond medical care. Faith and spirituality are among the tools that are being investigated.

As written earlier, faith is the substance of things hoped for and the evidence of things unseen. Faith is moving from the "invisible to the visible." James Fowler (1981) a Christian theologian, in his book entitled *Stages of Faith*, writes, "Faith is not always religious in its content or context." Faith, he adds, is a persons' or group's way of moving into the force field of life. It is a way of finding coherence in one's life and giving meaning to the multiple forces and relationships in that life. Faith is a way of seeing oneself in relation to others against a background of shared meaning and purpose. Paul Tillich (1951), in his text, *The Dynamics of Faith*, challenges readers to ask themselves what values have centering power in their lives. He iterates that the "God values" in one's life are those things that concern one ultimately. Real worship and true devotion direct one toward the objects of ultimate concern. That ultimate concern may finally center in one's ego or its extensions, work, prestige, recognition, power, influence, and wealth. One's ultimate concern may be invested in family, university, nation or church. Love, sex, and a loved partner may be another way to express one's passionate center or ultimate concern.

Ultimate concern is a much more powerful matter than claimed belief in a creed or set of doctrinal propositions. Faith, as a state of being ultimately concerned, may or may not find its expression in institutional or religious forms. Faith, so understood, is essential. It shapes how one's views life, how one invests in deepest love relationships, and their most costly loyalties. Thus, faith is a universal human concern (Tillich, 1957). Sometimes, however, faith and identity go into profound crises. This happens when the images of self are shaken and when one's very existence is challenged. In facing real or perceived vulnerabilities, one solicits faith in God, in others, or in the self. However, seldom is faith in self or others sought first. Faith in God, or a being greater than the human condition, is sought even though faith in self and others may also be desired. When faith in self or others is not forthcoming, one might feel abandoned by God. The perceived abandonment by God creates doubt, which in turn, may strengthen the faith in others. Some believe that they cannot be faithful until they have learned to be doubtful. Once there is clarity about doubt, there can be clarity about faith, particularly faith in God (vertical relationships), faith in others (horizontal relationships), and faith in self (personal relationships) (Fowler, 1981).

How then do faith and health interface? Faith and health interact at the point of relationships. There must be a relationship to define one's ultimate concerns in life (faith). They both go hand in hand, with relationships between the physical, social, psychological and spiritual dimensions of one's being, and relationships between the vertical, horizontal, and the personal dimensions of one's faith. When these relationships are out of synch and disconnected, invariably ill health and doubt occur (Fowler, 1981). One can be without physical disease, yet not be healthy, as in the case of mental illness. One can be without physical disease, yet have no purpose or goal in life and be hopeless. These are issues that need to be examined in order to determine health, quality of life and faith.

On the other hand, if one's relationship horizontally is off-centered, broken, and disconnected, can his or her faith be intact? Probably not. When relationships are repaired, then and only then can one move to being a whole and healthy person, having a faith that is strong, vibrant, intact and connected. It will take faith in operation, complimenting the other dimensions of life for a person to be healthy and whole. The goal is to bridge the spiritual dimensions of life with the other dimensions of one's being. Health promotion, in its conceptual sense, is empowering individuals and groups to address the ultimate concern of life: the physical, social, psychological and spiritual components of well-being in their physical and social environment. Ultimately, as biomedical research advances, less disease, sickness, and premature death will occur. However, health will not be reached until one's ultimate concerns are harmonized.

Health Promotion Strategies That Focus on Individual/Group Behavior

Everyone should have a good relationship with the health delivery system, which requires at a minimum, access to primary care. Individuals and groups must be in control of their health, not doctors. In fact, the training of health care providers to cure diseases often serves as a barrier to promoting health. To often the search for a cure bypassing simpler and more effective health promotion strategies (Warren, 1996). In other instances, the interventions needed are beyond the capacity or resources of the individual doctor or the health delivery system. Thus, rendering health care in isolation ineffective. For example, most of the previously listed morbidities and mortalities in the United States have social and behavioral risk factors. While the health outcomes may be heart disease, cancer, diabetes, or infant mortality, the risks factors associated with the causes of these diseases are social and behavioral. It is reasonable to believe therefore, that social and/or behavior interventions will more likely result in improved health outcomes.

In order to effectively intervene, health care professionals must place a greater emphasis on social and behavioral sciences. Figure 29 compares some of the tools needed for social and behavioral interventions versus medical interventions (Young, 1970). However, these needed tools have only recently been emphasized in the training of health professionals or in the provision of health care. The inclusion of religious practices and

	Medicine	Health Education Worker
Underlying Sciences	Physiology, anatomy, biology, physics, chemistry (to a lesser degree, behavioral science)	Behavioral Sciences: psychology, sociology, anthropology (to a lesser degree, natural sciences).
The Problems: Disease, dysfunction, illness and premature death	Physical illness, disease and dysfunction	Educational symptoms, e.g., need for regular care, failure to practice proper hygiene, poor nutritional practices, hopelessness, destructive behavior, low self-esteem.
Diagnosis Based on	Lab-Test, physical examination and observation	A person's or group's history of past experiences; information or knowledge levels; culture and traditions; personal or group goals; perceptions of doctors, health practice; life style and life circumstances.
Treatment	What shall it be? Who shall give it? When? Where? How?	Ibid. Evaluation.
Pharmacopeia	Drugs, radiation, prostheses, diet, et al.	Community organizations, films; group discussions; individual education; lectures; news releases; pamphlets; TV, et al., focus groups, faith community.
Follow-up	Periodic observations of symptoms, conditions and progress	Periodic evaluation of changes in knowledge, attitudes and behavior.

Figure 29.   Analogies between practice of dentistry and health education.

faith-based interventions in the training is emphasized even less (Furniss, 1994). The traditional medical model of care must be expanded to a faith-based model of care, which includes all the components of health: physical, social, psychological, and spiritual. The spiritual component is the foundation on which the other three components are based.

In order to fully integrate the social and behavior sciences and principles of faith and spirituality, the authors propose two health promotion approaches: one at the individual level, and the other at the group level. These approaches are not mutually exclusive. They obviously overlap, which may provide synergic effects.

At the individual level, five health promotion principles are recommended which include:

1. Eating the right food (i.e., nutrition and dietary issues)
2. Taking care of one's body (i.e., hygiene, exercise, and rest)
3. Getting along with others (i.e., interpersonal/social skills)
4. Protecting and respecting the environment (i.e., global planning), and
5. Believing in a divine order to the universe (i.e., spiritual grounding)

How can these principles prevent or reduce the impact of the major morbidity/mortality in the U.S. and abroad?

Eating the Right Food. The literature related to the role of nutrition and diet in maintaining health is quite strong. However, making nutritious food available and accessible has been difficult. Issues of poverty, preference, and cultural barriers require nutritional and dietary interventions well beyond the scope of today's health delivery system. Moreover, when the most nutritious foods are available and accessible, acceptability issues based on religion, beliefs and culture remain (Bass, Wyatt and Powell, 1982).

Taking Care of One's Body. The individual barriers that interfere with this principle continue to challenge the individual, group and health professionals. Again the literature is quite strong related to hygiene, rest, exercise and health (Carter, 1988; Ornish, 1984; Null, 1988).

Getting Along with Others. The most challenging example, which demonstrates the importance of this principle, is violence. The leading cause of death among African Americans (15–24) is violence. Increases in homicide and suicide are mounting in all segments of the population. While violence is the most obvious example, increases in mental illness, particularly depression, represent great challenges to behavioral health specialists, psychologists, and psychiatrists (Rutler, 1998).

Protecting and Respecting the Environment. As growing challenges to global health evolve, more and more evidence suggests toxic and hazardous chemicals and other environmental contaminants are threatening public health (Johnson, 1999). Increasingly, the health delivery system is being required to expand its capacity in environmental and occupational medicine. However the ability to respond effectively to these challenges is limited.

Believing in a Divine Order to the Universe. Distinguishing between religion and faith, and using these constructs in health interventions is increasing. This principle encourages the use of faith to enhance healthy living, healthy relationships, hope and expectation. These behavioral constructs are referenced more and more in the science literature as enhancing well-being and the quality of life. These health promotion principles are not meant to replace or minimize the value of the medical system. However, the principles will reduce the risk and adverse impact of the major causes of morbidity and mortality. More important, the principles are a part of a health promotion formula for well-being. While one cannot control all the factors that influence health, there are many factors that can be controlled by the individual, but are not being effectively employed.

At the group level, Chissell (1993) has developed an approach to health promotion called "Optimal Health." In his book *Pyramids of Power*, he discusses his transition as a physician, from providing "sick care" to "health care." In the Optimal Health paradigm, Chissell focuses attention on an ancient African-centered approach to Optimal Health. Interestingly, his approach is best suited for African Americans who continue to experience the greatest burden of disease and premature death. Optimal Health uses as its foundation, the following components:

1. Emotional health
2. Intellectual health
3. Physical health
4. Spiritual health
5. Socioeconomic health

He defines these health components collectively as "aliveness" and describes in detail the following activity necessary to obtain Optimal Health:

1. Optimal Emotional Health. Optimal emotional health involves managing the emotions to maintain joy, peace of mind and harmony within one's self as related to the environment and nature—all of the living things in one's world. In this state, one must feel by seeing, hearing, touching, smelling and tasting, but also with the higher facilities such as intuition (sixth sense), memory, visualization, imagination, faith, and trust.

2. Optimal Intellectual Health. Optimal intellectual health requires being aware of all thoughts, and choosing to actualize the thoughts that will move one toward his or her greatest potential and highest goal. Chissell writes that ancient African philosophers realized that thoughts are forms of energy—thoughts are things. Good thoughts, therefore, can enhance the probability of good things, such as health. Conversely, bad thoughts may worsen ones condition, or bring about bad things.

3. Optimal Physical Health. The three basic areas in Optimal physical health are Optimal rest, Optimal nutrition, and Optimal exercise. In this area, Chissell reminds the reader that in nature everything is relative and interdependent. Human beings must focus on these three components daily to sustain Optimal physical health. The body, he writes, is the "vessel or vehicle that contains our soul, spirit and personal spark of the Creator." He reminds the reader that in nature everything is relative and interdependent, and that Optimal physical health "feels so good." This area is usually the major focus in Western medicine.

4. Optimal Spiritual Health. Optimal spiritual health is the ability of every human being to believe in "Divine Intelligence" that remains within each human being as a life force. Chissell clearly separates Optimal spiritual health from religion. Meditation is recommended as one activity to enhance this connection.

5. Optimal Socioeconomic Health. This state of aliveness is related to coinhabitants of the immediate and more extended environment and how they contribute to one's self and others. The act and the reward of giving help to promote Optimal socioeconomic health. This area addresses ways of overcoming barriers, with enablers such as education, employment, and interpersonal relationships.

With these states of Optimal Health, Chissell expertly addresses issues of relationships to self, sexual intimacy, racism, economic development and other social constructs, which may result in adverse health conditions. The book unifies all the Optimal Health components and reintegrates them in an African context, directing the reader—particularly an African American reader—toward physical, social, psychological and spiritual well-being at both the individual and group level.

While these two health promotion approaches have been conveniently divided into individual and group approaches, they both have overlapping values. They are described separately because optimal health has far broader utility than the five health promotion principles. Nevertheless, one can use, both approaches synergistically. Both strategies consistently focus on positive behavior, minimizing disease and dysfunction, and optimizing all the components of health and well-being. They both emphasize social and behavior constructs such as hope, belief, will, and faith as foundations for health.

Health promotion is positive and not reactive. It searches for opportunities to affirm that which is good, and attempts to persuade individuals and groups that they can and should take control of their health and well-being. Health promotion addresses the quantity of life (how long one lives) and more important, the quality of life. How long and how well one lives must be balanced if Optimal Health is to be obtained. Health providers have a major role to play when the individual or group deviates from the principles of health promotion. The health care provider must intervene at the individual level, and public health officials must intervene at the group, community and population level. It is difficult to promote health when acute and chronic diseases and dysfunctions are rampant and go untreated. Leavell's "levels of prevention" complimented by Chissell optimal health paradigm, is the ideal overall strategy.

Significance and Expected Issue

To enhance health, one must clearly use social and behavior interventions in the best possible way. Some of these interventions are applicable to scientific inquiry, while others will be far more difficult to replicate or validate. For the researchable constructs, the following modified public health approach is recommended.

Defining the Problem

Through social and behavioral epidemiology, the practitioner's first task is to describe the problem, looking not only for problems, but also for enablers. He or she should seek what is right, as well as what is wrong. The patient is doing *some things* right. For example, how does one convince persons living in urban areas to reject the bad habits that accompany the "fast life?" Behaviors such as eating fast food rather than fresh, home-cooked meals, and not exercising are characteristics of urban living. People who live in rural areas usually exercise more and eat fresh foods because many have gardens. They eat better because fast food is more difficult to obtain. How do researchers convince people to adopt the advantages of urban life, while simultaneously rejecting the disadvantages? Social and behavioral research can help answer these questions. Public health interventions must encourage positive health behavior as well as discourage negative behavior.

Reviewing What Has Been Done

One can use the scientific literature and the popular media, and ask those who have the problem, especially those who are most burdened, what they think should be done. They may recommend a direction worthy of scientific inquiry or pursuit. Most people seek alternative advice in addition to professional medical advice and care. Friends, relatives are often asked for their advice about health. They can be helpful in identifying both positive and negative health behaviors at the individual and community level.

Developing an Action or Research Plan and Analysis

Using all the science available, the health care provider can gain insights from the biomedical, as well as the, social, cultural, anthropological and other behavioral sciences. True and equal partnerships must be developed with those that are being researched, for optimal outcomes.

Sharing the Results and Evaluation

All measures of success are not outcomes; process measures are also important. Focus on the population, in addition to the individual is useful. The subject should be the individual and the group. While the analysis must be valid and reliable, one must also value descriptive information. Unexpected positive consequences and social constructs are also noteworthy, even if they are anecdotal.

Discussing the Results

A discussion of what works, and what does not work is valuable. One must admit the limits of science, and acknowledge the art of healing. This awareness will enhance greater opportunities for Optimal Health. Some qualities have value, yet not measurable, such as hope, faith, and love. Empowering others by explaining to them the importance of their effort is essential to their continuation of that effort.

Sharing the Outcome and Acknowledging Both the Statistical and Practical Significance

Practitioners must insist on a broader view of health, and reject the separation of physical health from social, psychological and spiritual well-being. All of the components of health must be pragmatically targeted with the technology available. One must always recognize that these elements in isolation do not represent health. One must move from curing and preventing disease to promoting health at the individual, group, community, national, and global level.

Summary

Ultimately, "public health" means far more than a healthy body. It results in a well-adjusted individual, in a well-adjusted community, in a well-adjusted society-a global village in a perfect universe. If the universe was created perfectly, then human beings must learn to align themselves with the universe and all that it has to offer. However, health professionals, including social and behavioral scientists, and other human services professionals, must start where the people are. Many are sick, suffering and dying unnecessarily. Many are at great risk because they are low-income, undereducated, or live in isolated areas. Many are disproportionately ill because of racism, sexism, homophobia, and other behaviors that are discriminatory and unjust. This is the social context from which health and human services professionals of all types must work. This social context is, in fact, where health must evolve. The paradigm has shifted to not only include biological organisms attacking individuals, but to also include global changes, which threaten the existence of all humanity.

The Latin translation of the term science is simply "to know." Research is the method that science uses to know more. The goal of research is not only to answer questions, but also to raise new ones. Therefore, the authors raise the rhetorical question "What is health?" The answer is health is a relationship! Health and other human services professionals must eliminate or reduce the barriers to health and enhance the relationship between self and others, other entities in the universe, and the spiritual or religious principles. They must envision the ideal health outcome, design a plan of action, work tirelessly on that plan, believe in the outcome and expect a miracle. Miracles, large and small, happen every day.

References

Al-Faruqi and Ismail Raji, Eds. (1974). *Historical Atlas of the Religions of the World* (p. 209). New York: Macmillian.

Al-Faruqi and Ismail Raji, Eds. (1974). *Historical Atlas of the Religions of the World* (p. 73). New York: Macmillian.

Al-Faruqi and Ismail Raji, (1982). *Tawhid.' Its Implications for Thoughts and Life*, Wyncote: International Institute of Islamic Thought.

Al-Faruqi and Ismail Raji, Eds. (1974). *Historical Atlas of the Religions of the World* (p. 141). New York: Macmillian.

Al-Faruqi and Ismail Raji, Eds. (1986). *Trialogue of Abrahamic Faiths* (Herndon: International Institute of Islamic Thought).

Al-Faruqi and Ismail Raji, Eds. (1974) "Preface," *Historical Atlas of the Religions of the World*. New York: Macmillian.

Ali, Yusuf. *The Meaning of the Holy Quran*, Chapter 2, Verse 163–164. Ali, Yusuf. *The Meaning of the Holy Quran*, Chapter 7, Verse 42 Cohn-Sherbock, Dan. (1999). *Judaism*, NJ: Calmann and King Ltd. p. 20.

Ali, Yusuf. *The Meaning of the Holy Quran*, Chapter 50, Verse 16.

American Journal of Public Health, November 1999, Vol. 89, No. 11, p. 1645.

Asian, Adnan. (1998) *Religious Pluralism in Christianity and Islamic Philosophy*. Richmond: Curzon, p. 3.

Bass, B.A., Wyatt, G.E., and Powell, G.J. (1982). *The African American: Assessment, Treatment, and Research Issues*. NY: Grune and Straton.

Berger, P., Berger, B., and Kellner, Hansfried. (1973). *The Homeless Mind: Modernization and Consciousness*. NY: Random House.

Bloodworth, Venice (1979). *Key to Yourself*. New York: Devorss & Co.

Buchsbaum, Herbert (1993). "Islam in America," *Scholastic Update* (vi 26, n4), pp. 15–16.

Carter, A. (1988). *The New Miracles of Rebound Exercise*. AZ: ALM Publishers.

Chadwick, Owen. (1995). *A History of Christianity*. London: Weidenfeld and Nicholson. p. 202.

Chissell, J. (1993). *Pyramids of Power: An Ancient African Centered Approach to Optimal Health*. Baltimore, MD: Positive Perceptions Publications.

Choi, T., Greenberg, J. (1982). *Social Sciences Approaches to Health Services Research*, Ann Arbor, Michigan: Health Administration Press.

Chopra, D. (1989). *Quantum Healing: Exploring the Frontiers of Mind/Body Medicine*. New York: Bantam Books.

Chopra, D. (1995). Publishing, Inc. *Creating Health*. Canada: Random House Audio.

Chunn, J., Dunston, P. and Ross-Sheriff, F. (1983). *Mental Health and People of Color*. Washington DC: Howard University Press.

Cohn-Sherbock, Dan. (1999) *Judaism*. NJ: *Calmann and King Ltd*. p. 96.

Collins, Hall and Neuhaus. (1998). U.S. Minority Health: A Chart Book, NY: The Commonwealth Fund.

Covey, Stephen R. (1989). *The Seven Habits of Highly Effective People*. NY: Simon and Schuster.

Culle, M.R. and Rosenstock, L.M., (1998). "The Challenge of Teaching Occupational and Environmental Medicine." *Arch Inten Med* 148, pp. 2401–2404.

De La Carcela, V., Chin, J. and Jenkins, Y. (1998). *Community Health Psychology Empowerment for Diverse Communities*: NY, Routledge.

Fowler, James W. (1981). *Stages of Faith*. San Francisco: Harper & Row.

Fuchs, V. (1974). *Who Shall Live?* New York: Basic Books.

Furniss, George M. (1994). *The Social Context of Pastoral Care: Defining The Life Situation*. KY: John Knox Press.

Giorgi, E. (1974). "Community Medicines Relationship to Community Dentistry in the Delivery of Health Services, FNC. "Dummett (Ed.) *Community Dentistry: Contributions to New Directions*, Springfield, IL: Charles C. Thomas.

Healey, John W. (1997) "When Christianity and Buddhism Meet." *Commonveal*.

Hellberg, H. and Makela, N. (1994). Health For All or Some for Only (?) In K.S. Lankinsen, and Teal. (Eds). *Health and Disease in Developing Countries*. New York: Mcmillian.

Hick, John and Hebblethwaite, Brian, Eds. (1981). *Christianity and Other Religion*, Philadelphia: Fortress Press pp. 174–177.

Institute of Medicine (1999). *Toward Environmental Justice: Research Education and Health Policy Needs*. Washington DC., National Academy Press.

Johnson, B. (1999). *Impact of Hazardous Waste on Human Health*. New York: Lewis Publishers.

Johnson, B.L., Williams, B.C., and Harris, C.M. (1992). National Minority Health Conference Focus on Environmental Contamination. Princeton, NJ.

Keown, Damien (1996). *Buddhism: A Very Short Introduction*. London: Oxford University Press, pp. 13–15.

Kerting, F. (1973). *Foundation of Behavioral Research*, 2nd Ed. New York, Holt, Rinehart and Winston, Inc.

Leavell, H. and Clark, E. (1965). *Preventative medicine for the doctor in his community*. NY: McGraw Hill.

Lybarger, J., Spengler, R. and DeRosa, C. (1993). *Priority Health Conditions*. Springfield, VA: National Technical Information Service

Mahoney, Michael. (1999). "The Meanings and Correlates of Spirituality: Suggestions from an Exploratory Survey of Experts." *Death Studies* (v23 n6), pp. 521–528.

McCord, E. and Freeman, H.P. (1990). "Excess Mortality in Harlem." *New England Journal of Medicine*, October pp. 463–466.

National Center for Health Statistics, Health United States, 1998. *With Social Economic Status and Health Chart Book*. Hyattsville, Maryland.

Needlemen, H. (1990). *The Quiet Epidemic: Low Dose Lead Toxicity in Children*, Presented at the Charles A. Dana Awards Presentations for Pioneering in Health and Higher Education.

Null, G. (1988). *Gary Null's Complete Guide For Healing Your Body Naturally* New York: McGraw Hill.

Omish, D. (1984). *Stress, Diet, and Your Heart*. New York: Signet Books

Peck, Scott, M. (1978). *The Road Less Traveled*. New York: Simon and Schuster, pp. 167–168.

Roemer, M. (1976). *Health Care Systems in World Perspective*. Ann Arbor, MI: Health Administration Press.

Rogers, J.A. (1947). *World's Great Men of Color*. New York: Helga N. Rogers.

Ruffler, T. (1998). *Terra Infirma*. Harvard Public Health Review, Spring, Summer.

Rutler, T. (1998). Harvard Public Health Reviews. Spring/Summer.

Saleem, Shezad. *www.renaissance.com.pk*

Schrire, Carmel (1984). *Past and Present in Hunter Gatherer Studies*. London: Academic Press Inc. p. 231.

Sigerist, H. (1940). *Medicine and Human Welfare*. New Haven: Yale University Press.

Sigerist, H. (1946). *The University at The Crossroads*. New York: Henry Shuman.

Tamehill, A. (1985). "What is Health Promotion?" *Health Education Journal*; 44.

Taylor, S. (1993). In I. Vanzant (Ed.) *Acts of Faith: Daily Meditation for People of Color*. New York: Simon and Schuster.

Te Velde, Herman (1995). Theology, Priest and Worship in Ancient Egypt, *Civilizations of the Ancient Near East* New York: Charles Scribner's Sons p. 1746

Terris, M. (1992). "Concept of Health Promotion". *Journal of Public Health Policy*, 13(3), 267–275.

Tillich, Paul (1951). *Systematic Theology*, Volume 1. Chicago: The University of Chicago Press.

Tillich, Paul (1957). *Systematic Theology*, Volume 2. Chicago: The University of Chicago Press.

U.S. Department of Health and Human Services. (1985)."Report of the Secretary's Task Force on Black and Minority Health" *Executive Summary*. Washington, DC: U.S. Government Printing Office.

U.S. Department of Health and Human Services. (1998). *CDC Fact Book 1998*. National Center for Health Statistics.

Walker, B., Goddwin, N. and Warren, R.C. (1993). "Environmental Health and African Americans: Challenges and Opportunities." *Journal of the National Medical Association*. 85, 281–288.

Warren, R (1999). *Oral Health for All: Policy for Available, Accessible and Acceptable Care*. Washington, DC: Center for Policy Alternatives.

Warren, R. (1996). "Oral Health. From Cure to Prevention." Paper Presented at 10th International Associations for Dental Research Conference. Arusha, Tanzania.

Warren, R. (1997). "Assuring Oral Health in the Midst of Disease and Disability." Paper presented at the 6th World Conference on Preventative Dentistry: Capetown, South Africa.

Young, M. (1970). Dental Health Education. "*International Journal of Health Education*. 13(1), 1–26.

Chapter **10**

Healing an Addiction through a Twelve-Step Program Ending in Faith

GEORGE LANEY, GREGORY ROGERS, AND RICKY PHAISON

Introduction

There are no final answers to life's questions. As recovering addicts, we sought a way to live that offers continuing renewal rather than a once-and-for-all cure. We have been given the assignment to write about the process that has helped save our lives. This assignment is more difficult than it appears, because there is no official interpretation, which can be passed along.

The information here springs from our failure to come to terms with our addiction. For it is through the experience of addiction and God's grace this opportunity is afforded. Based on our experience, we believe that we suffered from an incurable disease of body, mind and spirit. We were in the grip of a hopeless dilemma, the solution of which is spiritual in nature. Therefore, this chapter will deal with spiritual matters.

We need to make an important disclaimer. This chapter presents our personal experience of healing an addiction through a 12-step program (Figure 30), ending in faith. In no way are we speaking for, or authorized to represent, any 12-step programs.

Being fallible human beings, our grasp of the twelve steps is incomplete at best. We hope that some of the information in this chapter will be helpful in the arena of public health, to the professionals in the field, and the recovery community. As you read this chapter, take for yourself the information you find helpful, and leave the rest behind.

We present this practical guide to the twelve steps, the process, and a path to the discovery and development of faith. The steps have provided us with a framework to give shape and direction to the many facets of our growth.

The nature of this process, the barriers, the internal conflict, and stumbling blocks were part of this process. The truth is, this process works because it saves lives and restores sanity. This is about an encounter with spiritual principles, which affect the individual.

1. We admitted that we were powerless over our addiction, that our lives had become unmanageable.
2. We came to believe that a Power greater than ourselves could restore us to sanity.
3. We made a decision to turn our will and our lives over to the care of God, as we understood Him.
4. We made a searching and fearless moral inventory of ourselves.
5. We admitted to God, to ourselves, and to another human being the exact nature of our wrongs.
6. We were entirely ready to have God remove all these defects of character.
7. We humbly asked Him to remove our shortcomings.
8. We made a list of all persons we had harmed, and became willing to make amends to them all.
9. We made direct amends to such people wherever possible, except when to do so would injure them or others.
10. We continued to take personal inventory and when we were wrong promptly admitted it.
11. We sought through prayer and meditation to improve our conscious contact with God, as we understood Him, praying only for knowledge of His will for us and the power to carry that out.
12. Having had a spiritual awakening as a result of these steps, we tried to carry this message to addicts, and to practice these principles in all our affairs.

Figure 30.   Twelve Steps of Narcotics Anonymous.

How It Was

The first mistake many of us make is, we think drugs are the problem. Drugs are only a symptom of a much deeper problem, which is addiction. To get a better understanding of addiction, we must look at the disease concept of addiction. From this point of view, addiction is a disease of attitudes and personality, featuring a general negative outlook that is rooted in fear, insecurity and low self-esteem. The main ingredients of addiction are obsession and compulsion. Obsession is a fixed idea that takes us back, time and time again, to our particular drug, or some substitute (anything that makes us feel good and gives instant gratification, such as money, power, sex, food, anger, etc.), to recapture the ease and comfort we thought we once knew. Compulsion can be defined as once having started the process with one fix, one drink, or one substitute, we could not stop through our own power of will. We were not willing to surrender control, which made us out of control and completely in the grip of a destructive power greater than ourselves. We had the ability to minimize or exaggerate our behavior, and denial was our constant friend.

Addiction is destructive and very insidious. It causes an internal disconnection of the human spirit, and expresses itself in ways that are antisocial. It dominated our thinking, emotions, and our actions in ways that cut us off from the outside world. It caused us to isolate, be hostile, resentful, self-centered and self-seeking.

Another aspect of our addiction was our inability to deal with life on life's terms. We developed a point of view that enabled us to pursue our addiction without concern for our own well-being or the well-being of others.

Our addiction put us in bondage. We were prisoners of our own mind and were condemned by our guilt of being dependent on a substance, to the extent that our ability to function was impaired.

History of the Twelve Steps

Twelve-step programs were born in the mid-1930s, with the establishment of the first program, Alcoholics Anonymous. Alcoholics Anonymous was adapted from a Christian revival organization referred to as the Oxford Group.

The spiritual lineage of the Oxford Group and AA runs through all of the movements of the Church beginning with Peter and Paul, and the other apostles who had a spiritual awakening, or renewal, as their goal. This was true through the various monastic movements, the Protestant Reformation, and the Oxford movement of the early 1800s. It was true, also, of the Oxford Group (originally called "A First Century Christian Fellowship"), an evangelistic movement of the 1900s, out of which twelve steps grew. Both the Oxford Group and the Twelve Steps have, at their hearts, the desire to take a healing message to people caught in unwholesome lifestyles.

Dr. Frank Buchman, a Lutheran minister of Pennsylvania Dutch stock, was the founder of the Oxford Group. This was the parent Group of Alcoholics Anonymous, which, in turn, is the source of the 12-step recovery process.

While attending the 1908 Keswick Convention in England, Buchman had an experience that changed his life. Bearing resentments and feelings of ill will toward the official board of a hospice he had established, and from which he had been compelled to resign because of differences with those board members, he entered a little church in Cumberland. His pride and anger had prevented his serving as a Christian minister should. Suddenly, in that church, through a woman talking about the Power of Christ's redemption, he envisioned the suffering face of the crucified Christ. In that moment, he realized the distance his resentments had placed between himself and God's unconditional love. Spiritually transformed, he was filled with an intense feeling of life as he surrendered his will and willfulness to God. The Oxford principles of surrender, restitution, and sharing were founded on his personal experience of spiritual conversion.

Later, Dr. Buchman worked with the YMCA in Pennsylvania and conducted evangelistic work in China. He gained some following through a series of revivals at Princeton, Yale, Harvard, Smith and Vassar, and kindred groups arose in Oxford and in other schools in England. Although Dr. Buchman and his following were later banned from Princeton and some of the other campuses, the group continued to reach out to the suffering through house meetings, which included testimonies, personal witness, Bible study, and informal talks. Members were encouraged to find and work with persons who suffered from problems similar to their own; for example, recovering alcoholics were encouraged to minister to others who suffered from alcohol dependencies. The use of attention-getting, easy-to-remember, easy-to-repeat slogans also became common in Group circles.

Bill Wilson, the founder of Alcoholics Anonymous, traced his journey to sobriety through the Oxford Group. In November 1934, while he was still a practicing alcoholic, an old friend, Ebby Thatcher, who had been restored to sobriety through the Oxford Group, visited Bill. One month later, while in a hospital undergoing treatment for alcoholism, Bill was again visited by Mr. Thatcher; at which time the principles of the Group were explained.

For the next three years, Bill Wilson pursued his recovery through the Oxford Group, which emphasized the following:

1. Complete deflation (of false pride)
2. Dependence and guidance from a Higher Power
3. Moral inventory
4. Confession
5. Restitution
6. Continued work with other suffering persons.

In the meantime, during a business trip to Akron, Ohio, Bill experienced a strong urge to drink. Fearing he was going to relapse, he began calling churches and asking if there was an alcoholic in that town with whom he could talk. He knew, as a principle of his Oxford Group activity, that he could only retain his recovery if he were actively involved in helping others like himself. The man with whom he was finally linked was Dr. Bob Smith, an alcoholic surgeon. They first met in May 1935, and Bill shared his own life story and his newfound spiritual realization that if he persisted in his drinking, he would either go mad or die. Bill and Bob talked night after night. Dr. Bob finally began to share frankly with his new friend. After ten days of sobriety that ended in one final binge, Dr. Bob had his last drink on June 10, 1935. Many people point to this date as the actual founding of Alcoholics Anonymous, although the group would not be known by that name for another four years.

In August, 1937, Wilson broke away from the Oxford Group, because certain alcoholics had trouble with its rather aggressive evangelism.

Despite this organizational break, the Oxford Group and the scriptures remained the foundation for much of Alcoholics Anonymous, and the Twelve Steps used in recovery programs today.

For us, recovery started with accepting the fact that we could not safely use a mind- or mood-altering chemical, and we had to stop using. In order for healing to take place, we had to go through the process, which took us out of the wilderness. This was our first free-dom from active drug addiction. In the framework of this step, our behavior change took place through surrender to the drugs, and a change in our attitude toward using drugs. This step promoted the new belief of accepting the cold, harsh truth that our drug-using career was over. The surrender that we gained in this beginning step opened us up to believe that our lives could change, and that God would place people in our lives to help us change.

Behavior change came about through our changed attitude toward drugs. Internally, we had to surrender, to the drugs and to this truth: if we continued our relationship with drugs, we would die. This is an internal change made possible through admittance and acceptance. We had to admit that we had a problem within ourselves that was magnified or intensified through active use of drugs. Making this admission brought us out of denial. So the price of admittance, along with abstinence was that we surrendered to this process, and through surrender, started believing that our lives could change. This was an internal move that had to be accepted on a deep level. We turned to our Higher Power and asked that the obsession to anesthetize or medicate our pain be lifted. The cooperation needed from us was to pray, go to meetings, and not to pick up any drugs. We needed to remem-ber: abstinence is the ticket that got us into the show, but abstinence is not the show itself.

Another part of this healing process began with self-acceptance, surrender to the self, as, the self is. Surrender was neither defeat nor a loss of power. It was a relinquishing of control. To surrender was to relax our grip on our former belief system and the life it bred. With surrender, we yielded to the change process, thereby gaining the freedom to change. The conflict that came when this belief system was questioned internally was stress producing, and frightening because it killed the lie that allowed us to look at our lives externally, not internally, to continue a relationship with drugs that was destructive and very insidious. This was the ending of life through rebirth, renewal and the resurrection of a different belief system. This was a very painful start of the faith-producing process, because we were asked to make an internal change to a familiar way of thinking and behaving. When we were in denial, despite all the evidence that said we had, at best, lost ourselves, a trail of destructive behavior and a body that had been devastated by active drug addiction, something in our heads would not cooperate. Our thoughts were divided, and even though we had fallen to the gutter, we still didn't want to surrender control of a broken and destructive life. It was there, but we struggled to accept it; we were defeated, but if we let this relationship with drugs go, what would replace it? How could we live with all this stuff going on within us, when all the decisions we made were to avoid dealing with ourselves? It was painful to live with the drugs, and it was painful to live without them. We thank God for introducing us to a fellowship of men and women just like us, and using some of those people to assist us in the very beginning of our recovery process.

Under these conditions we were brought into the fellowship of men and women with a common problem. We had to connect ourselves to people so we could learn how to live without drugs.

We had to reach a point in our lives where we felt like a lost cause. We had no worth to our families, or our community. We had no marketable job skills. Failure had become a way of life, and anything dealing with self, be it self-worth, self-esteem, self-confidence, self-responsibility was not working. Any hope of getting better disappeared. Helplessness, emptiness and fear became familiar companions. We needed a change, because we felt like total failures. A change from that self-destructive system built on lies and cheating was needed, but how could we change? A power greater than ourselves introduced us to a process of change by bringing us to our first 12-step group meeting. We started on this road to recovery with the help of God; we were defeated, and didn't know what to expect. Our minds were working against us, saying we were not going to make it, but we gained hope from people in the Fellowship who said we could make it. Nobody told us this was going to be easy, but in time, we started thinking our lives could change.

The process began with the admission of powerlessness, which was in direct opposition with the addictive message. The addiction itself was telling us, more is what we needed, and we could handle it because of our high tolerance, even though the addiction creates long-term pain and discomfort. The central paradox of the beginning of this journey was that the admission of complete defeat actually became the foundation for the strength to overcome our dependency.

However, along with this admittance must come acceptance. In other words, admitting began the change in behavior, and acceptance permitted the change in our attitude toward drugs. Admitting and accepting powerlessness was vital to breaking the addictive cycle. We had to accept that the pain could not be erased or solved through the temporary anesthesia (drugs), which produced negative consequences of shame and guilt.

Understanding the addiction cycle is important because it helps explain why the admission and acceptance of powerlessness is the first step to recovery. Otherwise, we would have remained addicted. When we relied on our own thinking and will power, the only thing we knew to do was to self-medicate with drugs to remove the pain, but this escalated our addiction. Ending this cycle challenged us to do less, to yield, to surrender, to let go.

Modern understanding of addiction suggests that all addictions and compulsions are fundamentally shame-based. It has been proven that the shame feelings are produced in the family of origin. Addiction is distinguished by lack of freedom of choice.

First, in starting this journey to faith, we had to move beyond the fear of stepping off of the path of the vicious addictive cycle. The fear of withdrawal and the pain that went with it was one obstacle. This fear caused us an intense internal conflict in which we exaggerated the pain. The truth of the matter is, when an addict stops actively using, the mind and body conflict as they struggle to restore balance. However, greater than this physical struggle is the emotional and spiritual aspects of withdrawal from the addiction. The real fear in this case is probably the emotional fear of losing control. The paradox of this first step in this journey is the act of surrendering addictive control, which actually brings some stability.

Second, we had to break out of denial about our addiction. Denial blinded us to the reality of our addiction, and allowed us to travel the path of self-destruction through self-deception. In other words, we could lie to ourselves about the bondage of our addiction.

Denial and the cycle of addiction could not be broken without yielding to a power outside of ourselves. We surrendered because we were powerless, not helpless, over people, places and situations, and we learning to "let things go." The paradox of addiction is that the more we tried to compulsively control ourselves through the practice of the addiction, the more out of control we became.

For an addict, control or lack of it, is central to every aspect of life. To admit powerlessness is to align our human will to God's will so we can become the people God created us to be. In this first step, we admitted that we could not control our addiction and whenever we used a mind- or mood-altering chemical, it made our lives unmanageable. The key to working this step was to recognize that we had a problem, then acknowledge that we had tried everything we knew to solve the problem, and none of it worked. In essence, we honestly acknowledged that we could not solve this problem by doing the things we had learned how to do. Also, we could not do it alone. This next step was a natural outgrowth of the first, because we became open to the possibility that there was someone or something out there that was able to provide a way to help us stop using. At the core of the second step is the belief in some kind of Higher Power or God that could help us. The insanity of using drugs day after day while looking for a different result ended here. We realized that somebody or something could help us do something we could not do for ourselves. In order for us to go from brokenness to wholeness, we came to believe that God existed and were willing to search for Him. This is where we welcomed in a new life-giving source to restore us to wellness. Before we welcomed in a new power, we did some emotional and spiritual housecleaning. This is how we began our real recovery process and our spiritual growth. It was important that we stopped playing God for ourselves, got off our self-appointed thrones, and believed that we could be resurrected from the living death of our addiction, and that our lives could change. As we committed ourselves to a lifetime of recovery, we started to believe that there was a loving and kind life-giving force that loved us and was willing to place people in our lives to help us.

At this point we were not advanced enough in our faith to believe in this process, but God met us right where we were, and took us from there. In the beginning of this process we admitted that our lives were out of control and we were powerless to change on our own. Next we renounced every old God that we had worshiped (even ourselves) as powerless to save us, and looked to a new and loving Higher Power to restore us to wholeness. In time, we recognized God as that Higher Power and asked Him to assume control over and care of every aspect of our lives.

Step Three told us to trust in God, and we realized that the power that brought us to this point was still with us and would continue to guide us if we allowed it. The paradox of this step was that we were willful and self-centered or self-absorbed, but this often camouflaged a deep sense of insecurity and pain. This step invited us to get out of the center of our universe, and give that place back to God. Our concern with self created more pain, loneliness, and isolation. It was the progression of this disease that pulled us into its vicious cycle. This obsession with self eventually turned us against ourselves. In order to overcome this painful cycle with self, we had to step out of ourselves and look beyond ourselves. We came to the realization that we could no longer "drive our own cars." We had "driven our cars" in a self-destructive manner down a self-destructive path. Now we had to move out of the "driver's seat" and develop a new belief, one that went against our old belief system, which kept us from allowing someone else to take over the wheel.

This step forced us to make a decision, and our decision was based on new information. At first, we realized that someone could be our spiritual advisor, sponsor or close friend. As our recovery process continued and we grew spiritually, we realized that someone was God. With God's help we stopped trying to feed ourselves physically, emotionally and spiritually with drugs. Gaining freedom from the bondage of self was strengthened through our relationship with God. We began to make a conscious choice to meet our needs without the use of drugs. The key to getting out of the driver's seat was willingness. If we cracked the door just a little bit, then God was willing to direct us in the process. The door we had to crack could only be opened on our end. We turned the knob on a door that opened on our side and we invited God in. Willingness was the key, and when we opened the door, God's healing love impregnated our lives and we no longer had to stand alone or carry the whole load. On an emotional level, we gained courage, strength and hope to move ahead in our recovery through our decision to ask God for help.

Step three told us to trust in God because we realized that God's power had brought us to this point in our lives, and was still with us and would continue to guide us if we allowed it. The steps allowed us spiritual healing from a spiritual disease.

A searching and thorough personal inventory was crucial to understanding the new direction of our spiritual growth. Knowing the steps of our past journey helped us to honestly look at our present situation. An important counterbalancing dimension of our inventory included noting the positive, as well as the negative, things about us. This inventory was an honest self-appraisal. There was no new beginning if we had no way of ridding ourselves of the burdens and traps that controlled and prevented our growth in the past. We wrote about the confusion and contradiction of our lives. We put ourselves on paper and looked at parts of us that we were afraid of. We wrote to free ourselves of living in old, useless patterns, and to grow and gain strength and insight. It took courage and faith to look at the secret parts of our lives. But we did not do this alone, because we were connected to our Higher Power. All the previous step work was a foundation for this step of relief. We asked our God's help in revealing the defects that were causing us pain and suffering. We needed courage to be fearless and thorough. We were not perfect, and we needed to look at our weaknesses. In accepting our weaknesses we became strong. No longer did we have to walk around afraid to look at ourselves.

We needed to look at our vengeful resentments, self-pity and pride. We wrote about our twisted relationships with family, friends and our community. In most cases, this meant we had to examine our childhoods, the experiences or messages, negative or positive, about ourselves that we absorbed in our families of origin. This was a crucial part of our journey to faith and a better relationship with our Creator.

All of what we discovered about ourselves in our inventory was to be freely admitted to God, to ourselves, and to another human being in Step Five. This was the most challenging step we faced in our process, but it was the most fulfilling, because it removed us from isolation. We shared this step with a trustworthy, compassionate human being. The value of this step was (1) our shame was reduced through confession; (2) we expressed our grief, expelled the resentments, anger and fear that blocked our relationship with others and God; (3) We shared our deepest, darkest secrets and our most private hurts with another human being; (4) Addiction by its very nature, isolated us from other people and from God, sharing this broke down the barriers we had erected through our addiction. Confession or sharing was the beginning of the end of our isolation.

When we had completed Steps Four and Five, we had created for ourselves an honest, realistic, yet loving self-portrait. During the course of making this journey we were asked consistently to go against our belief system. Each step we took prepared us for the next step in the process. The first five steps had to be done before we came into a state of readiness. One of the potentially frightening aspects of working Steps Six and Seven was they required us to deal directly with God. We were left alone to communicate directly with our God, to look directly at our relationship with God in the privacy and brokenness of our own hearts and minds.

The primary message of Step Six was simply that God was in charge of our change. We had to understand that we did not make defects go away. The work that we had done up to this point allowed us to see that we were not perfect. The spiritual principle of Step Six was willingness. Being ready was a spiritual condition. This step was about learning how to sit still with ourselves as we were. Human willpower was not effective in changing character. To be present in our own character meant that we must accept help for amending our defects. Our defects of character caused us to act in self-destructive ways when we knew better. These defects caused us to suffer, because their demands weakened us. The reality was that most defects of character involved some imbalance in the expression and experience of our most basic human needs. God wanted us to progress in the building of character, and we needed willingness and openness. Steps Six and Seven were difficult for us, but they would have been impossible if we had not yet accepted the presence of a Higher Power.

It was not necessary to present ourselves to God in any other way than we actually were. We presented ourselves just as we were, because God's love was already ours through His grace alone. Grace is unmerited love and favor. It does not have to be earned or bargained for. It simply exists. Whether we believed this or not depended on our faith. We had to believe in something here, and if we lacked in our belief, it was an obstacle on our journey. Faith in a Power greater than ourselves was vital and a necessary part of this process. It was important to remember that as we developed and nourished faith in God, we needed to consciously cling to it on a daily basis. Working and living the Sixth and Seventh Steps was an ongoing process.

Just as a plant has to be watered again and again if it is to live, so does faith. It needs care and attention to remain strong and healthy. This lifelong process is just that—a process. Our hearts and minds had to be open and receptive to the deep internal changes that could only be brought about by God. What we had to do here rather than exert power and control over our defects, was to yield, step out of the way and allow God to work in our lives.

The recovery process is a series of deaths and rebirths. We died time and time again to the reliance on our old belief system. We had to continually give birth to new life that was spiritually oriented and filled with the love of God. In Step Six, we asked God to remove defects of character, and this removal required that we die to old ways of being and acting. We had to die to our dependency on mood-altering drugs or chemicals, as a means of satiating spiritual needs. The expression of God within us could only be alive to the extent that we had died to our old ways. Letting go of old dependencies was easier said than done. Each of us had to come to the point where we were truly committed to making that break with our past, no matter how painful the process. Such a break could take place only when we had become totally willing and ready for God to work radically in our lives. One of the greatest challenges of our human experience was to find a proper balance in the expression and the fulfillment of our God-given needs for love, security, and acceptance. Our addictive personalities caused distortion of these needs. Here we wanted to avoid two extremes: (1) the tendency to deny or suppress the existence of our God-ordained needs and (2) the tendency to over-express or over-fulfill these needs.

Any change in our way of dealing with life required that recovery be a spiritual process. The beginning, the progression, and the tragic end of this disease were at the core, spiritual, directly causing harmful consequences in our relationships. Relationships with people significantly deteriorated because the relationship with drugs was time-consuming and essential. The same thing happened in our relationship with God. There was a detachment from God, and a disconnection from the part of us that made us alive.

We asked for guidance so we could discover what needed to be done, and then asked for the inspiration to do it. Here we gained, through our personal struggle, a better understanding of who God was and how God operated in our lives. Our concept of God at three days clean was very different from our concept of God at three years sober. God did not change, but our understanding of Him did. While Step Six focused on our willingness to yield our flaws to God, Step Seven centered on the humility with which we should approach Him. We asked God to give us courage, the strength, and the means to do the work. We needed to continue in a positive direction, and the key was humility.

It was very important that we did not confuse *humility* with *humiliation*. God did not want to mortify us. He just wanted us to submit to Him. We needed an attitude in which we maintained a realistic view of ourselves and our place in the world. Also, we had to understand our role in our own recovery, appreciating our strengths and limitations, and having faith in God. Our addiction caused us to deny and minimize the pain our defects inflicted. In trying to assess our character defects, we had to take a humble approach to avoid underestimating their severity. Also, humility was needed so that we could acknowledge the limits of human power in addressing these character defects. Humility was needed so that we could appreciate the enormity of God's power to transform lives. It was humility that allowed us to see our dependence upon God. For without some degree of humility, we could not stay sober, live a sober life, or walk a spiritual path. Without some degree of humility we could not live up to a useful purpose, or, in adversity, be able to summon the faith that could meet any emergency.

The invitation to humility was not an invitation to low self-esteem or a negative self-image. In fact, quite the reverse was true. Low self-esteem could be camouflaged by a superficial sense of false pride and a resistance to God's intervention. In contrast, if we had healthy self-esteem we would be free to come out from behind our masks and receive and appreciate God's greatness. When our self-esteem had been restored to a proper state of balance, we were able to comfortably humble ourselves before Him.

As a word and as an ideal, humility was misunderstood. At one time we had no room for humility in our lives. Our everyday conversation highlighted the pride we took in our own achievements. It was *our* show, and we took credit for it. It was through the process that we realized only God could relieve us of the useless or destructive aspects of our personalities. We could not handle the ordeal of life by ourselves. Our primary focus of daily living had to be based on honesty, tolerance, true love of other people and God. The basic ingredient of all humility—a desire to seek and do God's will—had to become part of our lives. All of the Twelve Steps are based on humility. Another simple definition for humility is truth, which is the root of faith. For a firm belief in God demanded that we take someone else's word other than ours. We had to accept things on the word of God; we had to be willing to learn more about God, and humbly ask Him to remove our shortcomings. Without humility this was impossible.

God removed our shortcomings by empowering us to do what needed to be done in dealing with our problems. God, as we have mentioned, was the source of courage, strength and hope on which we centered our recovery. We moved out of our addictive frame of reference by turning to God for help in solving problems. God gave us serenity, the state of mind that allowed us to accept ourselves fully, as we were, in all of our strengths and weaknesses. Through serenity we believed our lives were unfolding as they should unfold. Here, we came to terms with the fact that God took over the job of rebuilding our lives in HIS WAY.

Although Step Seven was the shortest step in terms of wording, and perhaps the least discussed in the recovery community, it was probably the most potent of the twelve. It embodied the miracle of transformation as we turned over our broken, defeated personalities so God might mold us into healthy, effective instruments of His will. We were humbly asking God to remove from our lives those things that were damaging to us, to our relationships with others and to our relationship with Him. This discipline was difficult (grievously) in the short term, but as we continued to humbly acknowledge God's authority over our lives and submit to His leading, it became easier. We were rewarded. As we humbled ourselves before God as his children in need, God lifted us up by filling our innermost hunger. Our humble confession was we couldn't meet our needs by our own striving. Instead, we had to place our troubles in God's care. We had turned from trusting in ourselves to trusting and delighting in the power and strength of God alone.

A program of spiritual growth sounds intangible, mystical, and hard to get our hands on. But in many ways, the spirituality of the Twelve Steps was a foundation of stone and mortar that we could see, hear, and touch with our own hands. We were making lists, paying old or neglected debts, taking daily moments of quiet time during which we stopped all activity, being honest when evasion seemed easier, telling our story, and listening to others tell theirs.

The Eighth and Ninth Steps suggested concrete, deliberate actions. The goals of these two steps were our own peace of mind, and relief from shame and guilt.

Our purpose in Step Eight was to achieve freedom from the guilt we carried by repairing the things around us that were damaged by our addiction. The willingness to make a list of all persons we had harmed cleared away the fear and shame that our past held for us. We were ready to say good-bye to shadows. This step said, take a pencil and paper and make a list of the names of the people we had harmed and become willing to make amends to them all. When we put someone on our list, no further action was required at that time. It meant that we could honestly admit that our actions caused someone harm.

We made our list, or took it from our Fourth Step, and added additional people as we thought of them. These additional people included the ones who loved us, or, those whom we loved. We could not be a member of a family or live with someone without hurting them at times. Our active addiction put anyone we contacted at risk, and we had to include these people.

Here we began to end our isolation from others and healing lives that had been dominated by guilt. This was our step toward freedom from the toxic residue of shame that came about through our hurting of other people.

Step Eight asked us to suspend our own judgment, bitterness and resentments toward others. We were tempted to tell ourselves that we would make amends to others—if and when we knew they could reciprocate. The spirit of Step Eight, however, required that we be willing to make such amends *unconditionally*.

Having come to a knowledge of God's love for us and the necessity of our love for him, we learned that His will was that we also love our neighbor, and we endeavored to find out our true relationship with God.

For years we had gone on with the false attitude that our neighbor existed for our benefit, that we were the ones to whom all owed homage. Now we learned that we had obligations to our neighbor, and that all of these obligations were based on the primary law of all human relationships: we must love our neighbor as ourselves.

For years we carried around in our confused minds a very long list of the persons who, so we thought, were harming us. We had to replace that phony list with a true list of the persons we had harmed. First, we had to let go of all those former false notions of the many harms that were done to us. We had to let go of the deeply ingrained habit of blaming others and circumstances for our difficulties. We honestly admitted that we were responsible, and when we were harmed, we forgave the person for the wrong committed against us. We did not forgive other people in order to help them; we did it to help ourselves.

The action produced in Step Eight offered immediate benefits, and freed us to begin our amends in Step Nine. The making of amends is a very strong tradition in the Twelve Step community. We could not avoid this step, since it provided an opportunity to make things right. The important thing was to take action and be ready to accept the reactions of those persons we had harmed. Readiness to accept the consequences of our past acts and take responsibility for the well being of others at the same time was the essence of Step Nine. We made amends when possible, because they were supposed to be made. Amends allowed us to make sincere efforts to offer an apology for past harm. Amends were wonderful bridge builders for more positive future relationships, and effective agents for removing the tremendous weight of guilt, shame and remorse.

A clear difference between Steps Eight and Nine was that Eight included *everyone* to whom we were willing to make amends. In Step Nine, we used a high degree of discretion regarding those to whom we would make amends, and when this should happen. Timing was an essential part of this step. We could make amends when the opportunity presented itself, except when to do so would cause more harm. Sometimes we could not actually make the amends; it was neither possible nor practical. In some cases, amends were beyond our means. We found that willingness could serve in the place of action if we were unable to contact the person we had harmed. However, we could never fail to contact anyone because of embarrassment, fear or procrastination. We had to remember when making amends that we were gaining relief from our past. We accepted that it was our actions that caused our negative attitude. This step helped us with our guilt, and helped others with their anger. Sometimes the only amends we could make were to stay clean. We owed it to ourselves and to our loved ones. We were no longer making a mess in society as a result of our active drug addiction. Sometimes the only way we could make amends was to improve the quality of our lives and give something back to our community.

By its very nature, the amends process of Step Nine was one-sided. The people to whom we extended amends did not have to reciprocate by forgiving us for the hurt we had caused them. Nevertheless, from the spiritual perspective, casting off old bitterness and tendering amends was freeing and healing. Most people wanted peace in their lives, but many never knew the complete peace that was available to them because they were not willing to be true peacemakers.

Steps Eight and Nine were bridges to the restoration of healthy relationships in our lives. We knew that our actions, for good or ill, had enormous impact on those around us. The establishment of good human relationships required a delicate balance between giving and receiving, between meeting the needs of others and finding healthful ways to meet our own needs. Step Nine emphasized the making of amends to others as a corrective balance against the self-centeredness of our old way of living.

This process was about learning how to live. We were impregnated with the spiritual principles learned in the first nine steps, and through their application in our lives, we made it possible to live in harmony with others and ourselves. In conducting our lives on a spiritual basis, it was critical for us to examine ourselves, confronting what we found, and taking ownership of our wrongs. What happened was as we changed on the inside, it was reflected on the outside. As behaviors changed, our perception of ourselves changed. Our task, after becoming more visible to the outside community and ourselves was to maintain this progress.

The last three steps, Ten through Twelve were the maintenance steps. These last three steps repeated many of the principles in the previous steps, but emphasized the value of continuing our relationship with the steps on a day-to-day basis.

Step Ten encouraged the taking of a personal moral inventory, which for us as recovering persons, had to become a daily process. Our faith in this journey was strengthened here, because we continued our movement forward. We continued to move because it was through movement that this faith process was made manifest. Life continued, human growth continued, and spiritual development continued. We had to continue to free ourselves from the wreckage of our present. We processed life more quickly than before by promptly admitting our wrongs. If we made a mistake, we did not get hung up on guilt and shame; we faced what we had done, and made amends. This step allowed us to be ourselves and accept ourselves as human beings subject to error. Yet here we formed a habit of looking on a regular basis at our actions, our attitudes, our relationships and ourselves.

In order to continue on this journey sober, it was necessary to keep in our conscious mind that we were what we were by the grace of God. It was through God's grace that we made this progress, and we realized that all of his was a gift of God.

Here we had a continuation of Step Four, Eight and Nine. When we took our inventory we had a rude awakening. We thought we were big shots with a good business and no faults. But, when we took stock honestly, we found our perception was distorted. To prevent a relapse into our old twisted way of thinking, we took a daily inventory. In this inventory we did not pay very much attention to how we had succeeded, but only if we were honestly trying.

We ran the risk of falling into spiritual pride here. Spiritual pride was the result when we looked for our faults, but concentrated too much on our progress, which was dangerous. If, through God's grace, we were empowered or enabled to eliminate many of our faults, we were liable to take the credit ourselves. This was pride again, and pride always comes before the fall. So through humility, we were conscious of the fact that it was God's work, not ours, and that was how we avoided the pitfalls of spiritual pride.

For our own growth and development it was important that when we were wrong we promptly admitted it. If we did not, we would begin to think that the other person was at fault, and resentment would come in, grow, and bear the fruit of discontent, negative thinking and neglect of loving our neighbor. This continued inventory kept us in the proper perspective. If we habitually omitted this inventory, it was impossible to have a true knowledge of what the love of God and our neighbor demanded of us daily.

Our daily inventory needed to assess the status of our relationship with God, especially, since our need to surrender ourselves to God on a daily basis would go on throughout our lives. This step was needed in our process to maintain a fit spiritual condition. We knew that it was only through our relationship with God that we had been given a new life.

Responsibility was reinforced in this step. As we became more and more responsible for ourselves we took responsibility for our actions. It wasn't our past or our parents who were to blame for what we did; our troubles were of our own creation.

None of us ever reached the point where our old nature was completely subdued, and we were careful not to be tempted by old, destructive patterns of behavior. We had to acknowledge our dependence upon God rather than ourselves. When we began to experience some manner of success in turning our lives around, we knew these accomplishments had resulted from "God's power, not our own human power". This step helped us to "think soberly," which simply meant we had sound thinking about ourselves, which was essential to our spiritual and emotional well-being. In any failed attempt to handle a problem, we could honestly admit our error, and ask God's help to correct the situation. Our personal inventory helped us remain focused on who we were and the direction God wanted for our lives. We had to pray constantly, and when we did something that was harmful to our recovery, we tried to fix it immediately; this step acknowledged that we sought *progress* but not perfection in this effort.

Our experience with the first ten steps cleared the way for the Eleventh Step. We went through a lot of hard work with the earlier steps in this process, and it took a lot of practice. We found ourselves changing as we continued in the process. We came to see that this step was the motor that powered the process, because it provided daily spiritual maintenance. This was where we improved our spiritual understanding of God.

The stage has been set for us to improve our conscious contact with the God of our understanding. Our spiritual condition, at this phase of our development, was the basis that offered unlimited growth.

One of the things that were very hard for us at the beginning was to have a God to believe in and to pray to. But, by practicing these principles, we gradually came to believe in a Power greater than ourselves whom we could trust in and rely upon. It was through this connection that our relationship with God started to grow.

Over time we became comfortable with God, praying only for knowledge of His will for us and the power to carry it out. This led to an intimate relationship with God; we built trust by taking things to God in prayer. It was to God that we could take our daily inventories of grief and confession issues. One purpose of this step was to increase our awareness of God, and to improve our ability to stay connected to this source of strength in our lives.

It was easy to slip back into our old ways. To ensure our continued growth and development, we had to learn to maintain our lives on a spiritually sound basis. God did not force His goodness on us; we could freely receive it if we asked. We prayed when were hurting, afraid or worried. This step reinforced our decision to believe in a Higher Power, and to know that Higher Power was God.

It was through prayer that we communicated our concerns to God. It took us a while to see that we could never pray too much. Praying relieved us of the need to worry over our problems and control the outcome. When we prayed we felt reassurance, because we were acting on our belief trusting that God was the ultimate authority in our lives and that communication with Him was possible and necessary.

Here we made an honest effort to pray and meditate daily. We sought to improve our conscious contact with God. We could not stagnate and accept whatever idea of God happened to be ours at the beginning of his journey. Our open minds allowed us to accept the blessings we had received, and we knew they came from God. It was through the process we gradually became more and more God-conscious. We opened ourselves and prayed for knowledge of God's will and asked for the strength. This step let us know God was in charge, and we had to ask for His assistance daily. It was through praying we opened up to God's healing power, and as our faith grew, it encouraged us to continue our relationship with God and prayer.

For us, life had been an experience of looking for love, security, self-worth and peace. We thought we had gained it through drugs. Our whole life and thinking was centered in drugs. But we finally came to know God, who could satisfy us in our spirit, in a way that drugs could not. The quality of our emotional recovery was dependent upon the maintenance of our spiritual condition, and so the quality of our spiritual condition depended upon maintenance of close communication with God.

It was here through the spiritual channels of prayer and meditation that we connected with God. We knew without question our need for this connection because prior to recovery we were foolish, disobedient, deceitful, dishonest, and hateful. This connection allowed us to know our blessings were a gift from God.

Our search to know God more intimately through recovery was a journey. This faith journey was not easy. Daily we encountered rough roads of temptation. We had struggles and discouragements, but through trusting and obeying God we were strengthened. We continually acknowledged our dependence upon God for any successes we hoped to have in our lives.

Our commitment to total abstinence and to this way of life became stronger as our conscious contact with God improved. We found that God had a wonderful plan for us, which brought us out of the dark into the light. This was something better than anything we had conceived of before. We did not need to concern ourselves with self-centered wants and desires anymore because we had been given a new life.

One of the most fundamental principles in this process was to "Let Go and Let God." We let go of the obsessive and compulsive need to be at the center of our own universe. We let go of desperate efforts to function as our own higher power. At this point we had to let go of the need to be in charge through spiritual rebirth and awakening and we let God resume His rightful position as the centerpiece of our lives. As we sought spiritual solutions to the old self-destructive drive, we discovered God gave us knowledge to handle situations, which used to confuse us. We realized that God was doing for us what we could not do for ourselves.

When we began this journey, we suffered from spiritual malnutrition. We entered recovery to heal our addiction to drugs, and found that, in the end, we had received far more than a specific healing of addiction; we had received the gift of a profound spiritual awakening. In a sense, the addiction, the pain, the healing of the addiction had been only stepping-stones to spiritual transformation and renewal that led to faith, the knowledge that God is real.

The Twelve Steps opened us up to living and was our path to God. The spiritual awakening was a result of living the steps. The process allowed us to gradually come to believe that a power greater than ourselves could restore us to gradually come to believe that a power greater than ourselves could restore us to sanity. We, who were hopeless, found hope. In time, we became willing to make amends to those we had harmed. The result was that we found freedom. We went through the process and grew. We began to experience the elements of a spiritual awakening—hope, gratitude, humility, freedom from addiction, and faith.

Maybe there are as many definitions of spiritual awakenings as there are people who have had them. But certainly each genuine spiritual awakening has something in common with all the others. These things that they have in common are not hard to understand. Awakening meant that we now became able to do, feel and believe in a way that we could not do before with our unaided strength and resources. We were granted a gift, which amounted to a new state of consciousness and being. We were set on a path that let us know we were going somewhere, that life was not a dead end, not something to be endured or mastered. In a very real sense we were transformed, because we became connected to a source of strength that at one time we had denied. We possessed a degree of honesty, tolerance, unselfishness, peace of mind and love of which, at one time, we were incapable.

What we found was this spiritual awakening was an awakening of our *own* spirituality. It was a slow, gentle reviving of spiritual awareness. We had developed a spiritual way of life and found some peace of mind in the process. We came to see that a spiritual awakening was being aware that God was there, and this allowed us to accept life on life's terms.

Our awakening gave us a message to carry to others. Emphasis was placed on reaching out to those who still suffered. We "can't keep it unless we give it away." Having received healing and spiritual renewal, we retained them only as we offered them to others. The evangelism aspect of Twelve Step recovery provided a bridge that linked us to others. We who suffer from addiction and have found spiritual healing from it were finally in a better position to understand and help others with similar problems. All we could do was carry the message.

We had spiritually transformed, and people were observing it in our lives, in our relationships with others and God. Our transformation was apparent in all the arenas of our lives. Healing our addiction was not the only goal of recovery. Rather, it was the starting place that began the real journey of spiritual growth. Our lives had to be remade. We had to remember that this growth was a process in the directions towards faith and God. As we learned to practice spiritual principles in our daily lives, we saw positive results. But the most wonderful feeling we found was that of being a part of humanity after so many years of isolation.

Our new lifestyle, free of the destructive dependency of the past, was a living witness of God's power to resurrect. Sharing our stories and recovery experiences in meetings and in personal conversation was a powerful spoken witness. We had to faithfully tell others what great things God had done for us. We became vigilant, since the need for spiritual self-discipline never ceased. "But for the grace of God" had multiple meanings for us. "But for the grace of God" we could still be in the bondage of our addiction. "But for the grace of God," we might not have found God and been given the opportunity to be reborn to Him. Step Twelve was a grace-filled step. Having been ushered into a spiritual awakening, we were commissioned to radiate God's grace to those around us.

As our lives became focused on God, we never concealed our past. In sharing our previous life, we were able to show others just how merciful, gracious and patient God is. God used our triumphs over our past to glorify Himself. God placed before us opportunities to share how we had been changed.

All of the sacrifices of the first eleven steps had purchased a gift beyond measure: our spiritual awakening to the God of our understanding. We came into recovery to save our lives when we were spiritually bankrupt. We gained more than we expected; we had come to a new and intimate understanding of God that allowed us to become instruments of His healing in our community. As people in our community saw our new value, and the strength and love God had poured into our lives, the very way we lived in the community spoke for itself. As we told how God had transformed our lives, our word not only helped others, but encouraged our own spiritual growth as well.

Although we have depicted our journey through the Twelve Steps in past tense, it is important for us to state that this is an ongoing process that continues in the present, and for the remainder of our lives. We must continue to live this process in order to recover.

Now we show up in the world, present in the moment. We are visible without fear, without shame, without false pride. We get to be who we really are. This is self-acceptance.

We have learned to carry serenity within us, and so we move from the place of being loved and accepted to the place of being present for other people.

"Faith," as defined by Barnabas, "is the substance of things hoped for, the evidence of things not seen." It is the builder of the seemingly impossible. It is the evidence of God's promise fulfilled. Our privilege is to accept, use, develop, and enjoy the fruits of faith. Our recovery is a fruit of faith. Faith is victory for us. We know that all our development, physical, mental and spiritual, depends upon our faith in God, our own fellow man, and in ourselves. Just in proportion to the amount of faith we place in God and ourselves, just so great is our development.

Faith sustains us when everything seemed against us and we developed faith by the use of it. It cannot be taught or forced, neither can it be destroyed. Through the exercising of faith we are able to help others. Thus shall our faith develop and become real evidence of things not seen. We now show by our actions in our daily lives that we believe, that we have faith, and, that we know as we use what we have that more will be given.

In using the knowledge we have gained by knowing ourselves, in practicing principles, and in never letting our faith falter, we build, step by step, that which has become living truth in our lives and has given us the ability to make an impact on the lives of individuals with whom we come in contact. As we apply what we know, there is given a greater understanding of how faith increases and becomes a living thing in our experience. In our daily lives, we are reflections of what we worship. We let our light shine so that others seeing the light in us may glorify God.

Faith guides us in the journey and tells us how to go about traveling through life. It is the map of the trip, the road signs, and the instructions. It is, in truth, the condition without which we can't make spiritual progress, without which we can't make progress in life and in living.

When we can still hold on when the day is dark and the way is obscure, this is evidence that we have faith. We have come this far by faith, and gained the greatest gift anyone of has ever known: a second chance.

References

Basic text of Narcotics Anonymous. The Twelve Steps are reported with the permission of Narcotics Anonymous World Services, Inc.

Budman, S.H. (1999). *Forms of Brief Therapy*. New York: Guilford.

Gorski, T.T. (1989). *Understanding The Twelve Steps*. Englewood Cliffs, NJ: Prentice-Hall.

Jennings, P. (1991). To surrender drugs: A grief process in its own right. *Journal of Substance Abuse Treatment*, 8, 221–226.

Knight, G.A.F. (1983). *Psalms*. Philadelphia: The Westminister Press.

Martinez, Y. (1995). *From Victim to Victor*. San Diego, CA.: Recovery Publications.

Wright, H.N. (1993). *Recovering from the Losses of Life*. Grand Rapids, MI: Fleming H. Revell.

The Coauthors

Maurice Apprey, Ph.D., is Associate Dean for Minority Affairs, University of Virginia, School of Medicine, Charlottesville, Virginia, and Faculty Member, Center for the Study of Mind and Human Interaction.

Carl C. Bell, M.D., is President and CEO, Community Mental Health Council Foundation, Chicago, Illinois; Professor of Public Health and Psychology; and Director, Health Research and Policy Centers, University of Illinois, Chicago, Illinois.

Rena G. Boss-Victoria, Dr.P.H., MPH, MS BSN, is Associate Professor, Public Health Program, and Director, HIVIAIDS Prevention, Evaluation and Policy Research Center, Morgan State University, Baltimore, Maryland.

Jay Carrington Chunn, Ph.D., is Associate Vice President for Academic Affairs, Professor, and Principal Investigator, Public Health Planning Program, Morgan State University, Baltimore, Maryland.

Jimmy Cunningham, B.A., is Director, Violence Prevention Program (Office of Minority Health), Philander Smith College, Little Rock, Arkansas.

Brian Flay, Ph.D., is Professor of Public Health and Psychology; Director, Health Research and Policy Centers, University of Illinois, Chicago, Illinois; and Principal Investigator, Aban-Aya Project.

Marlene Greer-Chase, Ph.D., is Assistant Professor, Department of Teacher Education and Administration, Morgan State University, and Research Group Participant, Preventive Science Workgroup, Johns Hopkins University Prevention Center.

Lewis M. King, Ph.D., is Executive Director, Fanon Research Center, and Professor of Human Development, Drew/UCLA Medical School, Los Angeles, California.

George Laney, M.Ed. (Rehabilitation Counseling), is Project Coordinator, Research 3 Project, Johns Hopkins University School of Hygiene, and Twelve-Step Program Community Activist, Baltimore, Maryland.

Valerie Lawson, Ph.D., is Professor, Howard University, Washington, D.C., and Research Evaluator, Violence Prevention Program (Office of Minority Health), Philander Smith College, Little Rock, Arkansas.

William R. Lawson, M.D., Ph.D., is Professor and Chairman, Department of Psychiatry, Howard University Hospital and Medical School, Washington D.C.

The Reverend Harold C. J. Lockett, D.Div., is Ordained Minister, Church of God in Christ, and Associate Director for Professional and Pastoral Education, Life Link Foundation, Atlanta, Georgia.

Rolande Murray, Ph.D., is Assistant Professor, Department of Psychology and Rehabilitation Counseling, Coppin State University, Baltimore, Maryland, and

Prevention Science Specialist and Associate Science Director, Morgan State University Prevention Science Program, Baltimore, Maryland.

Roberta L. Paikoff, Ph.D., is Associate Professor, Department of Psychiatry and Psychology Institute of Juvenile Research, University of Illinois at Chicago, Chicago, Illinois, and Principal Investigator, CHAMP Project.

Ricky Phaison, is Addiction Specialist and Community Activist, Baltimore, Maryland.

Warren A. Rhodes, Ph.D., is Professor and Chairperson, Department of Psychology, and Director, University Prevention Science Program, Morgan State University, Baltimore, Maryland.

Gregory E. Rogers, M.Ed. (Rehabilitation Counseling), is Prevention Specialist and Counselor, Department of Education, Baltimore, Maryland.

Derald Wing Sue, Ph.D., is Professor of Counseling Psychology, Columbia Teachers College, Columbia University, New York, and President/Owner, Consulting Corporation in Psychology, Training, and Research, conducting research, training and consultation in multicultural psychology and education.

Rueben C. Warren, Dr.P.H., D.D.S., is Associate Administrator for Urban Affairs, Agency for Toxic Substance and Disease Registry, Health and Human Services (HHS). He is former Associate Director for Minority Health, Center for Disease Control and Prevention, Atlanta, Georgia.

Adnan A. Zulfiqar, B.A. (Religion and Anthropology), is Marketing Director for *Renaissance Islamic Journal*, Lahore, Pakistan, and Regional Research Assistant Trainee, Morehouse School of Medicine, Atlanta, Georgia.

Index

Aban-Aya, 18–20, 31, 33, 35
  community partnerships and coalitions, 22
  efforts to improve self-esteem, 29
  efforts to increase bonding and attachment, 27
  and health care, 24–25
Addiction, 153–155, 166–167; see also Twelve steps
  cycle of, 157–158
Adolescent risk behaviors, 106–107; see also Risk
  behaviors
Adult protective shield, reestablishing the, 32–34
Affinity bonds, 102
African American health problems, alternative
      models for viewing
  challenges, 95–97
  framework for authentic models, 101
  implications for, 97
  nexus of behavior change, 99–101
  parameters of culturecology framing, 101–108
  primacy of culture, 97–98
  reality of relationships, 98–99, 102–104
African American marginalization, negating, 96
African American youth
  health, 106
  violence among, 61–63
  violence prevention in, 63–64, 71
    Brother to Brother project, 64–71
African Americans
  cultural context, 101
  social structure and, 92–93
AIDS: see HIV/AIDS
Alcoholics Anonymous (AA), 155–156
"Aliveness," 146
Alternative medicine, 42, 46; see also Faith healing;
      Indigenous models of healing
Amends, making, 163–164
Anastamosis, 77
Asian-American mental health clients, 45
Assurance bonds, 103
Attachment, 25–28
Autonomous individual, idea of the, 100

Baltimore, priority problem areas in, 1–5
Behavior change, nexus of, 99–101

Behavioral change: see Health Behavioral Change
      Imperative
Behavioral disconnect, 6
Body, taking care of one's, 145
Bonding, 25–28
Bonds
  as basis of unity, 102
  four types of primary, 102–103
  health-enhancing and health-compromising, 103–
      104
Border crossing, threshold of, 80–81
Broken line, 77
Buddhism, 134

Caring, 121
Center for the Study of Mind and Human
      Interaction (CSMHI), 79–80
Change
  of function, 76, 84
  stages of, 99–100
Chicago Board of Education violence prevention
      initiative, 20, 31–34
  community partnerships and coalitions, 22–24
  efforts to increase bonding and attachment, 27–28
  and health care, 25
Chicago HIV Prevention and Adolescent Mental
      Health Project (CHAMP), 17–18, 29–32, 35
  community partnerships and coalitions, 21–22
  efforts to improve self-esteem, 29
  efforts to increase bonding and attachment, 26–27
  and health care, 24–25
Chicago Public Schools (CPS), 20, 22–23, 30–35
Christianity, 131, 132, 155
Chronic illness, 91–92, 129
Clarity, 121–122
Classroom management skills, need for, 57–58
Commitment, 122–123
Communal networks, 47–48
Communities, working with
  do's and don'ts when, 87–88
  need to know history of community when, 73–74
  public health practitioners, 114–116
Community Action Policing (CAP), 23

173

Community-based practitioners in public health, 123–124
Community-based prevention, 15, 22
Community epidemiology, 53
Community partnerships and coalitions, developing and expanding, 21–24
Community projects, 81
Connectedness dynamics, 25–28
Cultural context, 96–98, 101
Cultural memory
  modes of storage, 76–79
  sedimentation and reactivation of, 75–76
  transformation of, 84–85
Culturally framed events, 102
Culturally framed relationship, 102, 103, 109
Culture, 75–76; see also Ethnocentric monoculturalism
  defined, 75
  primacy of, 97–98
Culturecology framework, 101, 109
Culturecology framing, parameters of, 101
  basic assumption, 102–103
  case study, 105–108
  methodology, 104–105
  principles, 103–104
Culturecology intervention program, developing a, 105

Death, leading causes of, 137
Dehumanization, 78
Denial of addiction, 158
Development, life-course, 53
Diabetes, 104
Diet, 145
Difference and identity, 75
Differentiation, 80
Disease
  chronic, 91–92, 129
  concept of, 94
  in populations, 115–116, 118
Doctor(s) of Public Health, 114
  learning goals, 123
  role of the professional, 119
Doctor of Public Health (DrPH) degree program, viii, xi
Doctoral programs in public health, 113–114, 117; see also Public health practitioners
  changing scientific community-based instruction paradigms, 124
  community-based instruction, education, and behavioral change, 119–121
  elements for quality practice-based teaching and learning, 121–123
Doctorate in public health, 116
Doctors of Public Health, 116
Drug use, 11; see also Addiction; Twelve steps
DuBois, W. E., 99–100

Ecological perspective, 99; see also Culturecology framework
Emergency rooms, 8
Emotional health, 130
  optimal, 146
Environment
  and health, 128
  protecting and respecting the, 145
Epidemics, 129
Estonia, 79, 80, 82–87
Ethnic conflict, practitioners' need to have tools for solving, 73
Ethnocentric monoculturalism, 42–43
  overcoming, 44–45
Ethnonational conflict resolution, 74
Ethnonational conflicts, heuristic steps for negotiating, 79–80
"Eurocentric" public health approach, 100
Exercise: see Physical activity

Faith, 136, 168; see also God; Religion(s) and faith
  defined, 168
Faith healing, 128
Family networks, 47–48
Figure, 77
"Fixed position," 95–96
Fractions, differentiation within, 80
Function, change of, 76, 84

Gender differences in HIV prevalence, 4
Goal setting, strategic, 105
God
  conceptions of and beliefs about, 132–135, 143, 158–162, 164–168
  grace of, 167–168
Group networks, 47–48

Harmony bonds, 103
Health
  defined, 127–129, 149
  as dynamic interface, 127–128
  global threats to, 128–129
  in populations, 115–116, 118
Health behavior change, 99; see also specific topics
Health Behavioral Change Imperative, 5, 13–15
  as challenge for new millennium, 1
Health behavioral change imperative, and children, 73–75
Health behavioral change theory and practice dimensions, 10–13
Health Belief Model, 12, 100
Health care; see also specific topics
  community efforts to improve, 24–25
  defined, 117
  ethnocentric monoculturalism in, 42–45
  paradigm shifts in, 4–10
Health care administration, 117–118

Health care professionals, social and behavioral
    skills of, 143–145
Health care service provider roles, developing
    alternative, 45–47
Health care service providers, 8
    cultural competence, 43–44
    cultural flexibility, 46
Health professions, competencies and education
    needed by, 117–118
Health promotion, 141, 143
    defined, 96, 141
    principles of, 145
    strategies focusing on individual/group behavior,
        143–147
    vs. treating disease, 7, 114, 116–118
Helping relationships, cultural beliefs about, 45–46
Hinduism, 134
Hispanic persons, leading causes of death for, 137–
    140
Historical grievances, staging and transforming, 75–76
History, sense of, 75, 87
HIV/AIDS prevalence, and high-risk groups, 3–6,
    10, 13–14
    AIDS incidence and mortality, 4
Holistic outlook, 48
Hospitals, 8
Humility, 161–162

Identity, difference and, 75
Implantation, 77
Indigenous healing systems, facilitating, 47
Indigenous models of healing, learning from, 45–49
Indigenous support systems, facilitating, 47
Infant mortality, 138, 141
Information, new
    channels for, 123–124
Insurance, health
    persons without, 8–9
Intellectual health, optimal, 146
Intromission, 77–78
Islam, 132–133

Johns Hopkins Prevention Research Program (PRC),
    53–55
Judaism, 133

Klooga Project, 84–87

Language education, 82–83
Learning, 123–124
Life-course development orientation, 53
Line, 77
Locus of control, 130
Logan Square Neighborhood Association (LSNA), 23

Managed care, 7, 9
Medical model/paradigm, 93, 94, 99

Meditation, 166
Mental borders, crossing of, 80–81
Mental health care for racial/ethnic minority
    patients, 45
Mental health problems, 130; see also Emotional
    health
    prevention of, 52–53
Mental health professions, ethnocentric
    monoculturalism in, 42
Metal detectors in schools, 28
Minority groups: see Racial/ethnic minority groups
Modernity, 142
Moral inventory, personal, 164
Morbidity and mortality, trends in major
    and their social and behavior associations, 136–
    142
Morgan State University, vii, viii, xi, 8, 58; see also
    under Prevention science training program(s)

Narcotics Anonymous, twelve steps of, 154
Natural medicine: see Alternative medicine
Neuropsychiatry, 24
Nutrition, 145

Obligation bonds, 102–103
Optimal health (approach), 146–147
Other, the, 78, 80

Personal hygiene paradigm, 93, 95, 96, 99
Personal influence paradigms, 100
Physical activity, 11
Polarization, 80
Posttraumatic stress disorder (PTSD), 62, 63, 67, 69
Powerlessness, admission of, 157
Prayer, 166
Prevention, 7
    of disease, 118; see also Health promotion
    primary, secondary, and tertiary, 141
Prevention programs, categories of, 25
Prevention research science trainees, paths taken by,
    56
Prevention researchers, need for minority, 51
Prevention science, 51–52
    theoretical orientation for, 52–53
Prevention science framework, 53
Prevention science training program(s)
    changing face of undergraduate minority, 56–57
    Morgan State University's, 52–58
Preventive intervention approaches, 99–100
Preventive intervention trials, 53
Pride, 164–165
Project Hand-in-Hand, 82–84
Protection motivation, theory of, 100
Psychological genetic paradigm, 98, 99
Psychopolitical dialogue, 80–81
Psychotherapist-client relationship, cultural
    differences and, 45

Public health; *see also specific topics*
  as cultural phenomenon, 102
  culture of, 98, 102
  culturecology redefinition of, 105
  as the health of relationships, 97, 102
  major content areas of, 115–119
  meaning of, 149
Public health approaches/paradigms, 93–96, 147–148
Public health practitioners, advanced; *see also* Doctoral programs
  community-based, 123–124
  defining public health areas of knowledge for, 115–118
  need for new metaphor for, 114–115

Racial differences
  in health problems, vii–viii, 3, 5, 10, 41
  in mortality, 137–141
Racial/ethnic minority groups, disproportionate disease among, 129
Racial/ethnic minority patients
  health care for, 41–42, 45–46
  mental health care for, 45
Racism, 41
Rapid response teams, 34
Reasoned action, theory of, 12, 100
Recovery process, 161
Relationships
  getting along with others, 145
  reality of, 98–99, 102
  web of, 103, 104
Religion(s) and faith, 131, 136; *see also* God; Twelve steps
  belief in divine order to universe, 145–146
  concepts of, 131–136
  convergence of, 135–136
  and healing process, 48
  influence on health and health care, 142–143
  synergic relationship between health and, 130–131
Research, 105, 149
Responsibility, taking, 165
Risk, 98–99
Risk behaviors among youth, 10–11, 106–107; *see also specific topics*
Russians: *see* Estonia

Sanitation, 99
School-based interventions, 22
Schools, public
  level of discipline in, 57–58
Scientific rationalism, 94, 96
Self-acceptance, 156, 157
Self-efficacy, 12

Self-esteem, efforts to improve, 29–30
Sexual behaviors, high-risk, 10, 11, 21–22, 31
Sexually transmitted diseases (STDs), 4, 10
Shamanism, 47–49
Smoking, 6, 9
Social analysis, 115
  tools of, 115, 118
Social cognitive theory, 12
Social development curriculum (SDC), 19, 22, 27
Social learning theory, 11–12, 100
Social marketing, 13
Social skills, teaching, 30–32
Social structure, impact of, 92–93
Socioeconomic health, optimal, 146–147
Soviet Union: *see* Estonia
Spiritual awakening, 166–167
Spiritual health, optimal, 146
Spiritual pride, 164–165
Spirituality, 135–136; *see also* Religion(s); Twelve steps
  in being, importance of, 48
  defined, 135
Stages of change model, 99–100
Staging and transforming historical grievances, 75–76
Support groups, 21
Surrender, 156–157, 166

Teaching, redefinition of, 120; *see also* Doctoral programs
Technological advancement, and health care, 142
Theory of Triadic Influence (TTI), 19–20
Tobacco use, 6, 9, 11
Transgenerational haunting, 75, 77, 78
Transgressor and transgressed groups, 74, 77–79
Transtheoretical model, 99–100
Trauma; *see also* Posttraumatic stress disorder; Transgenerational haunting
  minimizing effects of, 34–35
Triadic influence, theory of, 19–20
Truancy prevention, 28
Twelve steps, 153, 154
  history of the, 155–168

Urban health, priority problem areas in, 1–5

Violence; *see also* Transgenerational haunting; *specific topics*
  exposure to, 62

Web of causation/web of interaction, 99
Wellness philosophy, 8; *see also* Health promotion

Years of potential life lost (YPLL), 136, 137